BOTANICAL TEAS RECIPE BOOK

Published by Herbal Academy
24 South Road, Bedford, MA 01731
Copyright © 2024 Herbal Academy

theherbalacademy.com

Text © 2024 Herbal Academy

Book Design:
Amber Meyers, Cover Design, Interior Design
Emay Allmendinger, Botanical Illustrator, Interior Design

Editors:
Amber Meyers
Jane Metzger, M.S.
Lindsey Feldpausch, RH(AHG)
Lisa Olson, RH(AHG)
Meagan Visser, BSN

Recipe Contributors:

Alison Birks, RH(AHG)
Alyson Morgan
Amber Meyers
Catarina Seixas
Christie Clark
Cristina Asensio-Foley
Felicia Cocotzin Ruiz
Greta Kent-Stoll
Hannah Lasorsa

Heather Wood Buzzard
Holly Hutton, RH(AHG)
Jane Metzger, M.S.
Jill York
Lindsey Feldpausch, RH(AHG)
Lisa Olson, RH(AHG)
Meagan Visser, BSN
Shona Richter MacDougall, RH(AHG)
Stacy Karen

International Standard Book Number
978-1-950671-05-2

Botanical
TEAS
Recipe Book

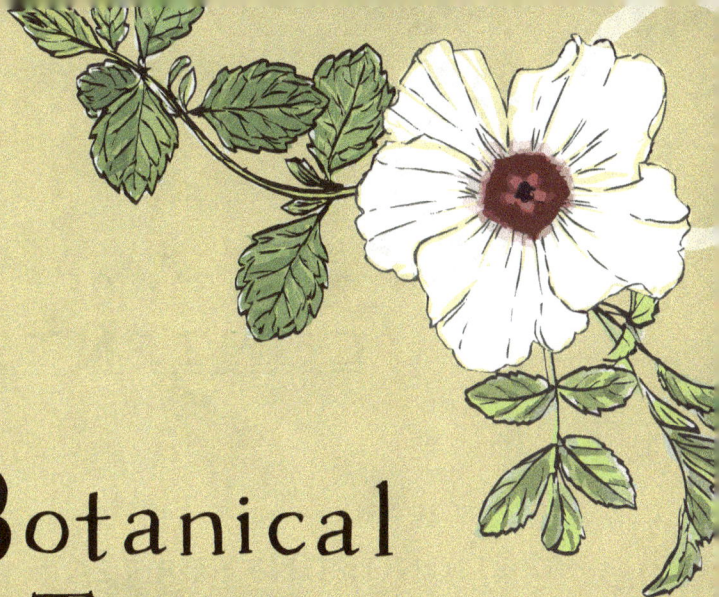

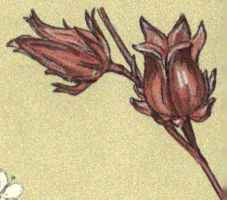

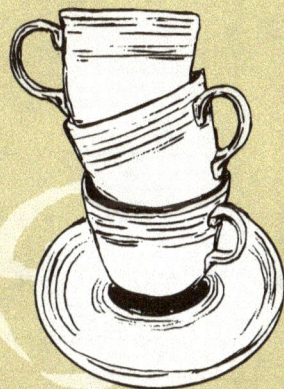

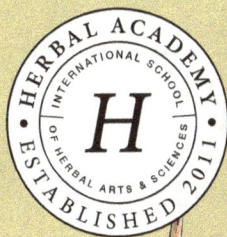

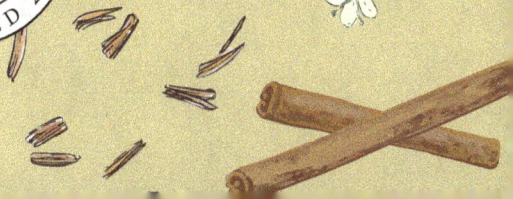

Herbal Academy · INTERNATIONAL SCHOOL · OF HERBAL ARTS & SCIENCES · ESTABLISHED 2011 · H

TABLE OF
CONTENTS

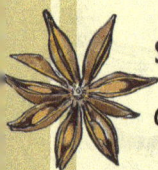

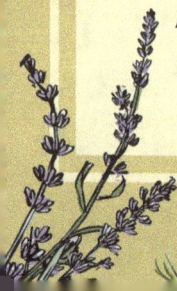

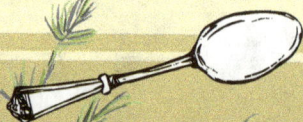

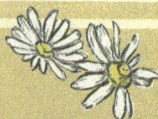

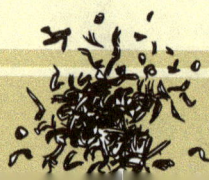

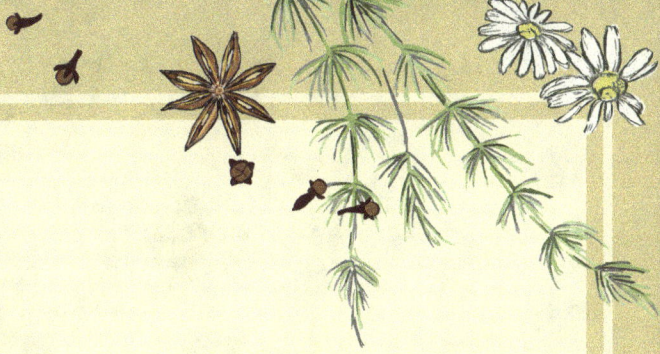

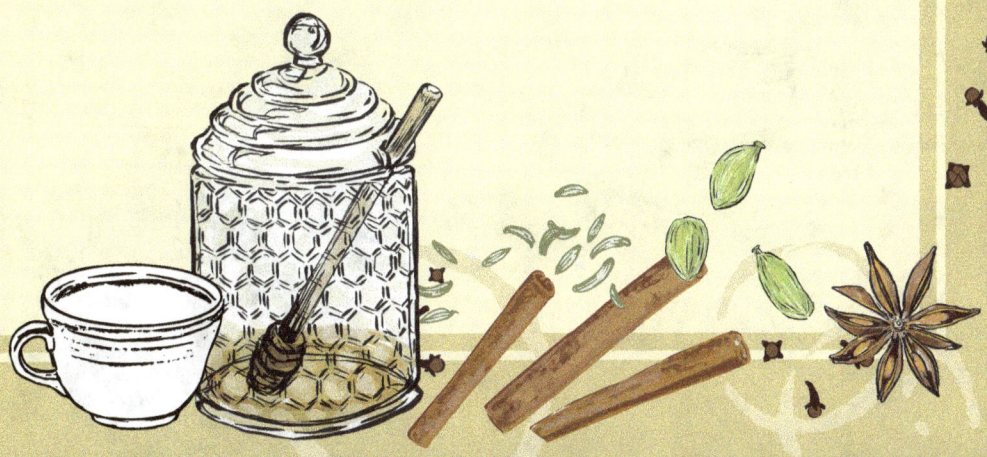

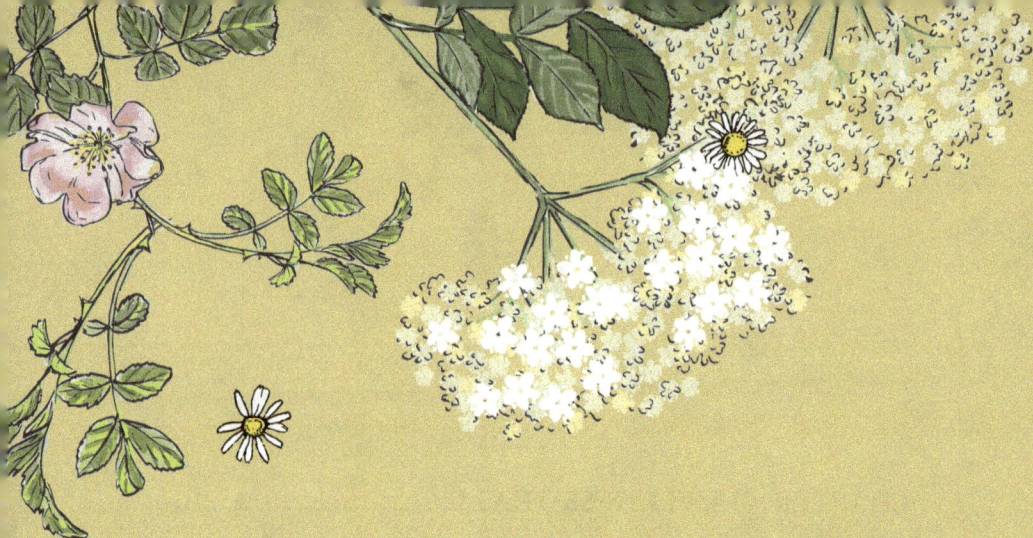

In memory of herbalist,

Herbal Academy Founder,

and very dear friend,

Marlene Adelmann,

who always had full teapots

to welcome us in.

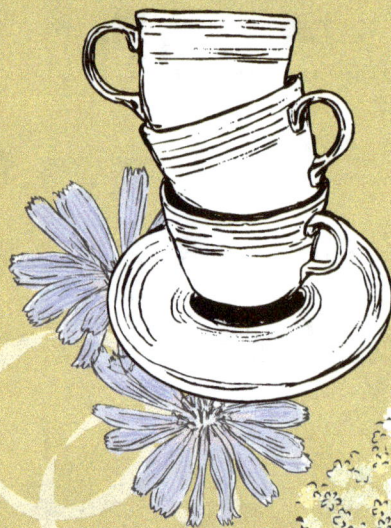

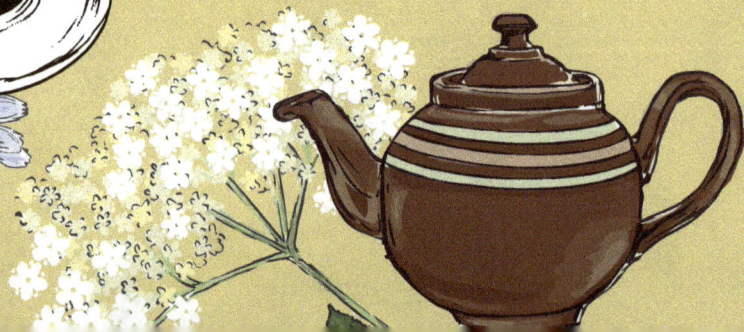

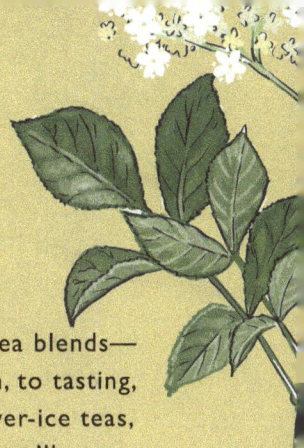

ACKNOWLEDGMENTS

As herbalists, we are passionate about botanical tea blends—from dreaming them up, mixing, and brewing them, to tasting, fine tuning, and sharing them. Give us hot teas, over-ice teas, sun teas, and bath teas (we'll take them all!), and we'll serve them in big jars, dainty cups, and on-the-go mugs morning, noon, and night. We love our herbal teas, made from a wide variety of botanicals, and they are our go-to preparations for so many reasons. Whether we're looking for flavorful hydration, a cozy moment with a warming sip, daily delivery of nutritive, mineral-rich herbs, support for acute symptoms or chronic imbalance, or connection with a plant ally, herbal teas can and do deliver! They are an accessible way to reap the benefits of herbs, and the process of preparing them is a nourishing ritual in and of itself that helps us slow down and feel connected with the plant world—and when shared, with each other.

The *Botanical Teas Recipe Book* is the third installment in the Herbal Academy Botanical Recipe Book Collection. We have long dreamed of creating this tea book for our community, and, now, in your hands, you hold a compilation of herbal tea blend recipes lovingly curated by the Herbal Academy team. We started this process in 2021 with the **Tea Blending 101 Mini Course** offered in our online classroom, with a set of 12 recipes intentionally focused on 12 commonly accessible herbs for maximum blending with minimum herbal input. Those original recipes and the well over a hundred more that you'll find in the pages to follow were masterfully crafted and curated from our personal notebooks and recipe boxes and taste tested to our satisfaction by the Herbal Academy team of Jane Metzger, Amber Meyers, Meagan Visser, Lindsey Feldpausch, and Lisa Olson with support from recipe crafters

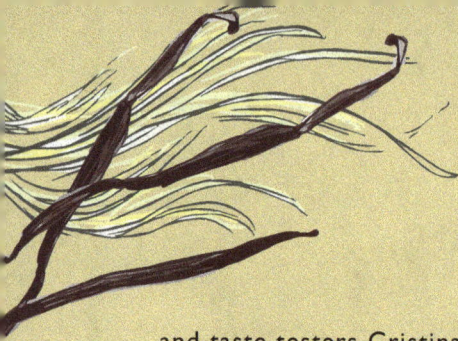

and taste testers Cristina Asensio-Foley, Alison Birks, Heather Wood Buzzard, Christie Clark, Holly Hutton, Stacy Karen, Greta Kent-Stoll, Hannah Lasorsa, Shona Richter MacDougall, Alyson Morgan, Felicia Cocotzin Ruiz, Catarina Seixas, and Jill York. Botanical illustrator Emay Allmendinger teamed up with Amber Meyers to create the beautiful drawings and book design to convey our love for plants and provide inspiration as we celebrate them in these treasured tea blends. Our heartfelt gratitude goes to this talented team who shares this passion for herbs, tea, and community!

Our wish is that this book and these recipes encourage you to bring herbal tea into the rhythms of your life, and that they not only become your go-to favorites, with dog-ears and dried tea splashes on the pages of this book, but our Herbal Academy favorite, time-tested recipes also inspire you to create your own personalized botanical tea blends through experimentation and adaptation.

As we so often say, it's always a good time for tea! Won't you join us?

Jane Metzger and Amber Meyers
Co-Directors, Herbal Academy

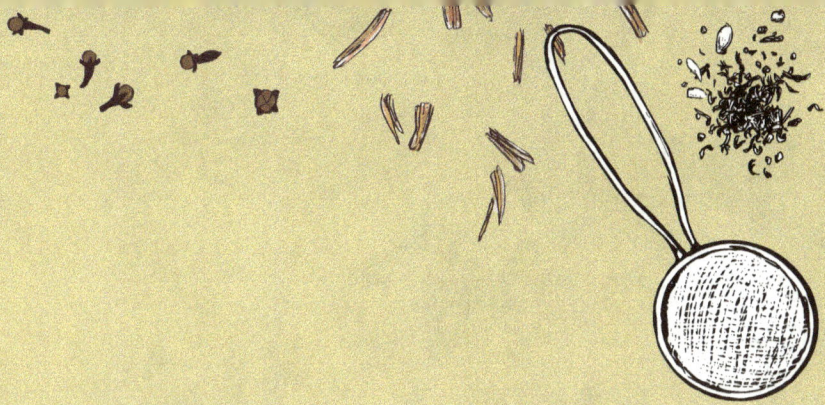

DISCLAIMER

While the herbs selected for these recipes are
typically safe in the suggested amounts for the
general population, always research the safety
of individual herbs in the case of particular
health conditions or during pregnancy
and lactation.

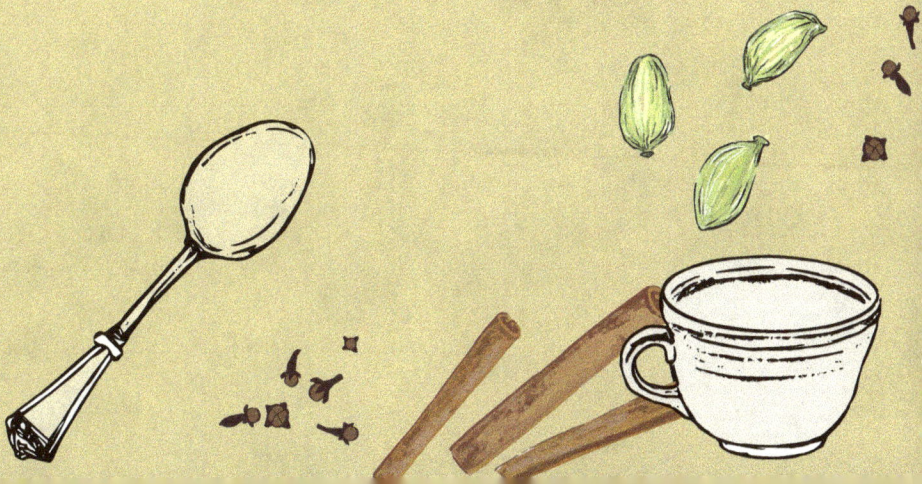

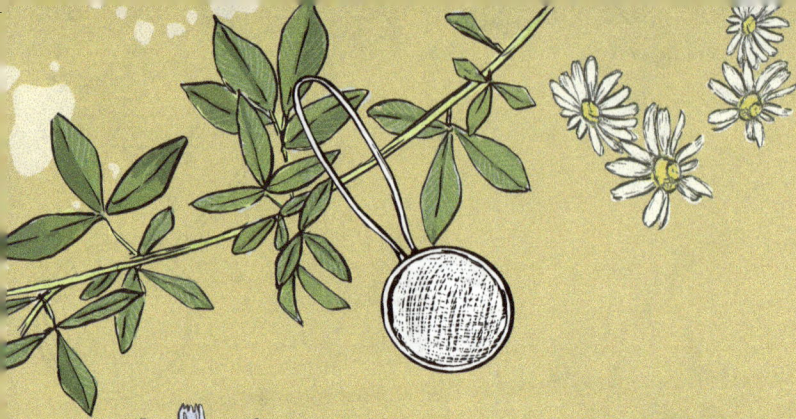

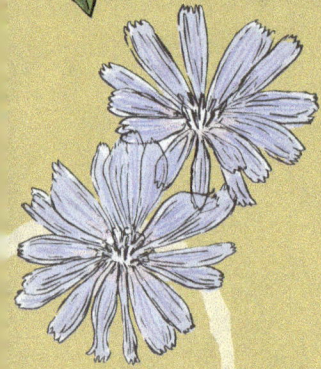

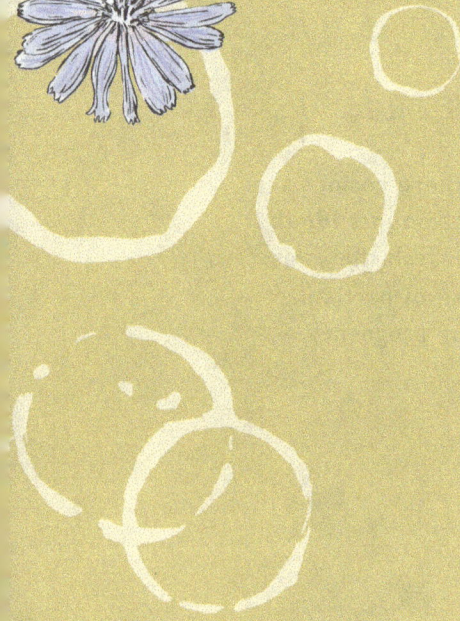

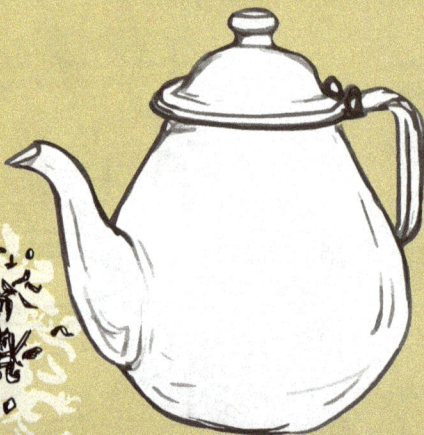

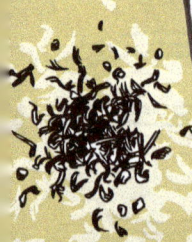

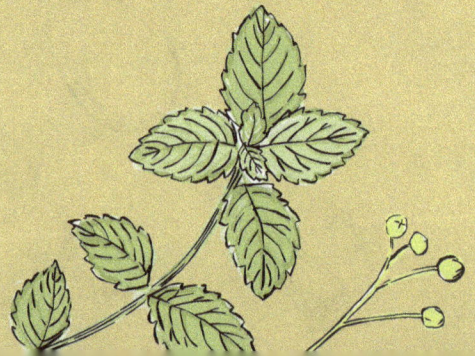

CHAPTER ONE
TEA BASICS

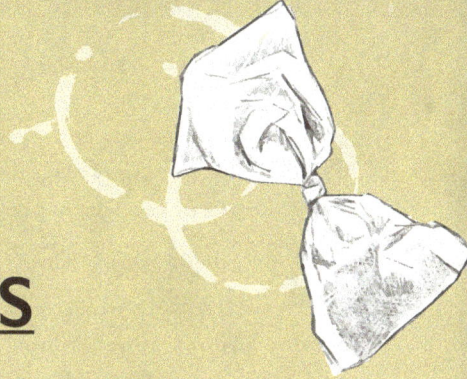

Whether you are making a single cup of tea for yourself, a lovingly crafted pot of after-dinner tea to share with your family, or a gallon of iced sun tea adorned with fresh flower garnishes for a gathering, botanical teas are always a lovely and supportive way to weave herbs into your routine. In this book, we have compiled an abundance of recipes to get you started exploring the wonderful world of herbal teas. You'll find blends inspired by the seasons of the year, blends for finding calm and encouraging sound sleep, blends that address acute concerns such as nausea and common cold symptoms, blends that support body system balance, and blends that offer a nutritive boost, just to name a few! There is something for everyone, with tea blends for simple delight as well as wellness-support blends that address the concerns many of us are familiar with.

But before we get to the botanical tea blends, let's back up a bit and learn about herbal tea and its benefits!

What is Tea?

Tea is a term you hear quite often, but it can have different meanings depending on where you're located or what's in your cup.

One essential thing to know about tea is that traditional tea, or *true tea* as some call it, is a water-based beverage made from the leaves of the tea (*Camellia sinensis*) plant. On the other hand, a water-based preparation made from the many other botanicals available in our gardens, meadows, forests, and grocery stores is typically called herbal tea. These botanical teas contain plant parts from various herbs, utilizing flowers, leaves, barks, roots, fruits, and/or seeds.

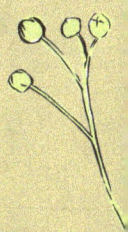

Even though you can certainly mix *Camellia sinensis* leaves with

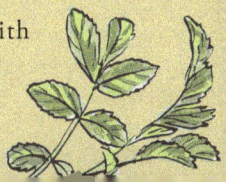

2

other herbal material, herbal tea is most often defined as tea that does not include *Camellia sinensis*, and in order to avoid confusion between the two types of tea, some people use the term herbal tisane when referring to a tea made without "true" tea.

Technicalities aside, we often use the term *herbal tea, botanical tea, herbal infusion*, or *herbal decoction* when talking about water-based plant preparations.

Benefits of Tea

Regardless of the term you use, botanical teas are wonderful beverages, and they come with many benefits for the mind, body, and spirit.

The first benefit that comes to mind is hydration! Whether you're sipping a cup of tea after dinner or drinking a quart of herbal infusion throughout the day, herbal teas are a great way to increase your water intake, helping the tissues of your body to stay hydrated.

Another benefit of preparing herbs as a tea is that the water you use to make your tea extracts the water-soluble constituents from the herbs in your cup—many of which contribute to the wellness-promoting properties of herbs! These constituents and their properties are then readily available to your body in a form that is easy to absorb.

In addition to the physical benefits tea provides the body, it is a wonderful support for the mind and spirit. Take for instance the way the warm cup feels in your hands, or the sight of the steam curling upward to caress your skin when taking those first sips. While the herbs you choose to use in your tea can help to soothe and calm you, taking notice of these sensory aspects of a simple cup of tea can be incredibly soothing and grounding as well.

One additional benefit is that making and drinking herbal teas is one of the easiest ways to begin using herbs. Not only are teas pleasurable to drink, but they're pretty easy to make without needing a lot of special equipment or preparation. Plus, the shelf life of teas is relatively straightforward—because you drink them up right away, preservation isn't as much of a concern as with other herbal preparations.

For all of these reasons, herbal teas are an excellent preparation to get to know and use regularly!

Infusions *and* Decoctions

While there are many similarities between infusions and decoctions, there are some differences—the biggest being the plant part used in the herbal tea blend and whether the tea is steeped or simmered.

INFUSIONS

An infusion is made by pouring hot or cool water over the leaves, flowers, and/or more delicate or aromatic parts of a plant so that the properties of the plant are infused into (extracted by) the water. These herbal preparations typically steep for 5-20 minutes, depending on the constituents of the herbal blend and the flavor you are looking for in the infusion, although sometimes they are steeped even longer.

For example, if you are making an infusion from a botanical tea blend that includes chamomile (*Matricaria chamomilla*) flower, chances are you will only allow this infusion to steep for 5 minutes. If it steeps any longer, the chamomile starts to taste bitter. On the other hand, if you are making a tea blend filled with mineral-rich herbs, like nettle (*Urtica dioica*) leaf, for example, you may want a longer steep time of 20 minutes or more (sometimes overnight!) to allow for optimal extraction of the nutrients.

That said, there are always exceptions to the rule. Some infusion recipes call for plant parts that are more difficult to break down, such as roots, barks, seeds, or berries, and these types of infusions can steep from 4-8 hours to overnight, as mentioned above.

If preparing an infusion from aromatic herbs rich in volatile oils, it is important to cover the jar, mug, or teapot during the steeping period in order to retain the volatile oils that are largely responsible for the flavor and aroma of the plant material as well as prepared tea, not to mention its efficacy.

Marshmallow (*Althaea officinalis*) root infusion provides another exception to the rule. Extracting this plant's moistening, cooling mucilage requires cooler water temperatures and a longer steep time, so a tea blend containing marshmallow root may need to steep in cold water for 1 hour or longer to best extract its beneficial properties.

4

DECOCTIONS

A decoction is made by simmering plant material in water over low heat, typically for 20 minutes or more, resulting in a concentrated liquid. Decoctions are used for tough and dense plant material like roots, barks, seeds, and fruits, which generally require more time and heat to break down for thorough extraction. These plant parts can often be decocted several times before being composted or discarded.

A classic decoction example is chai. Chai is made from hard plant parts (think cinnamon bark, fennel seed, and ginger root) and therefore needs a long steep time and more heat to best extract the flavors and plant constituents. Chai is traditionally made in India by simmering herbs in milk and water in a saucepan for 10 minutes or longer before straining the herbs, sweetening, and drinking. Many recipes also call for the addition of black tea (*Camellia sinensis*) leaf after the other herbs have decocted.

As mentioned above for infusions, when decocting aromatic herbs for teas, it is important to cover the saucepan with a lid while simmering to retain the volatile oils.

Now that you know about the benefits of botanical tea and the similarities and differences between herbal infusions and decoctions, let's look at some basic supplies you'll want to have on hand to make a cup or two of tea whenever you fancy it.

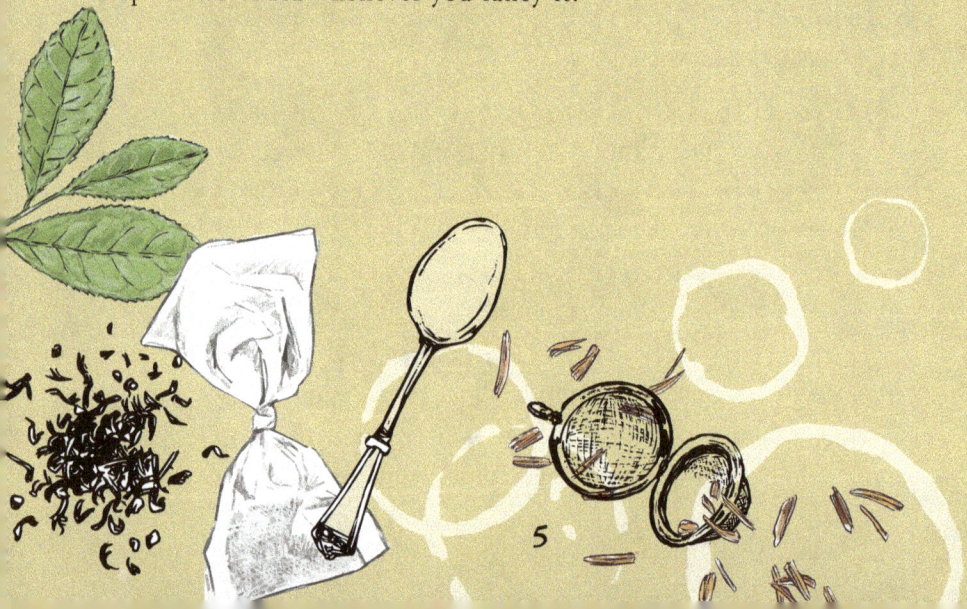

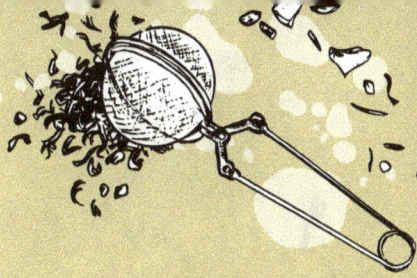

Basic Supplies

Whether you're making herbal tea a cup or kettle at a time, here are some basic items you may want to have on hand.

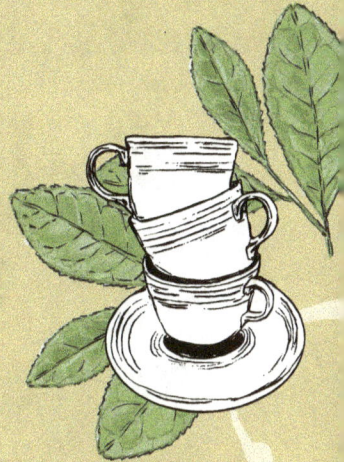

- Bowls (for blending herbs)
- Spoons (for stirring)
- Funnels
- Measuring cups and spoons
- Digital kitchen scale
- Spice grinder (for powdering herbs)
- Mortar and pestle (for crushing herbs)
- Saucepan, tea kettle, mugs, and tea strainers
- Labels
- Storage equipment, such as glass canning jars with lids, tea tins, and/or teabags

Once you've gathered all your supplies, you will be ready to make herbal tea blends and cups of herbal tea. But before we share our favorite recipes with you, we want to first give you some ideas on ways you can tweak or boost the flavor of an herbal tea blend when needed. Of course, it's always a good idea to try a recipe as written first to see how you like it, and from there you can adjust it a bit to make it your own.

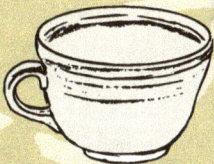
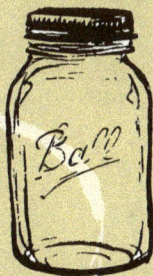
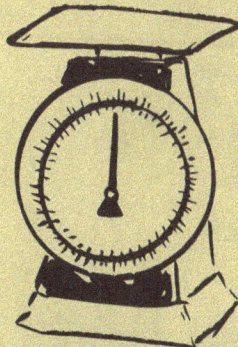
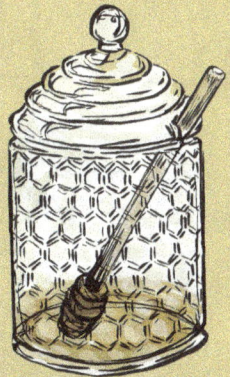

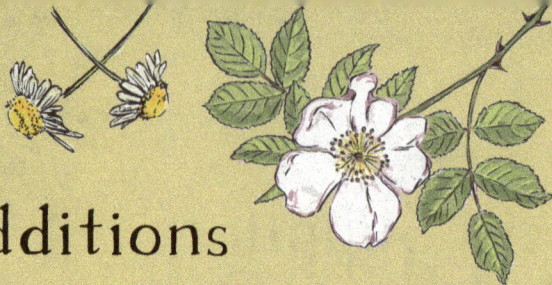

Tea Additions

Taste is important when it comes to herbal tea. No one wants to choke down an unpleasant-tasting tea, even if it's good for you!

Sometimes, the herbs that make up a tea blend will have enough flavor to make the tea palatable and pleasurable to drink. Other times, you may need to add additional herbs to achieve the deliciousness you desire!

With that said, it's important to rein things in to avoid including too many flavors in a tea recipe. If you're not impressed with the taste of a tea, try to focus on adding 1-2 flavors that will pair well with the current flavors of the tea, such as adding a fruit and a spice, lavender and vanilla, or a mint medley, instead of overloading the blend with four or five flavorful herbs.

If you decide to level up the flavor of a tea recipe, take some time to think about what herbs or other edible ingredients would enhance the blend's flavor or aroma. Herbs like chamomile (*Matricaria chamomilla*) flower, cinnamon (*Cinnamomum* spp.) bark, fennel (*Foeniculum vulgare*) seed, and peppermint (*Mentha* x *piperita*) leaf can help to add a lot of flavor and scent to a tea blend, as will dried fruit.

While there are many flavorful herbs that can be incorporated into tea blends, below is a list of 20 of our favorites.

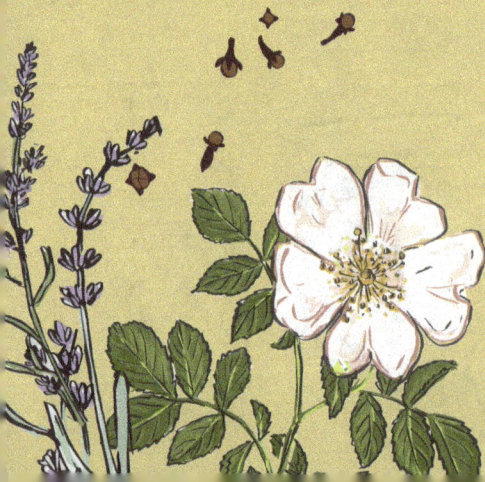

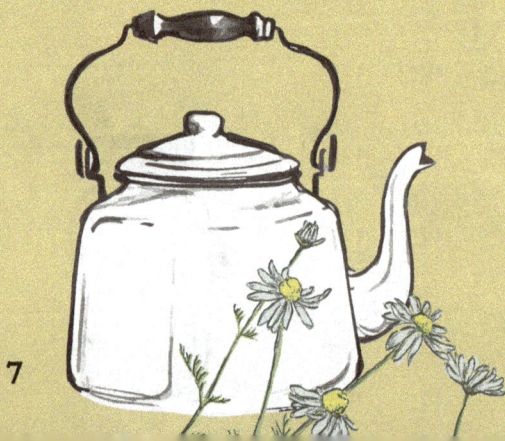

20 FLAVORFUL HERBS *for* TEAS

- ANISE (*Pimpinella anisum*) seed
- CARDAMOM (*Elettaria cardamomum*) seed and pod
- CHAMOMILE (*Matricaria chamomilla*) flower
- CINNAMON (*Cinnamomum* spp.) bark
- CLOVE (*Syzygium aromaticum*) bud
- FENNEL (*Foeniculum vulgare*) seed
- GINGER (*Zingiber officinale*) rhizome
- HIBISCUS (*Hibiscus sabdariffa*) calyx
- LAVENDER (*Lavandula* spp.) flower bud
- LEMON BALM (*Melissa officinalis*) aerial parts
- LEMONGRASS (*Cymbopogon* spp.) leaf
- LICORICE (*Glycyrrhiza glabra*) root
- PEPPERMINT (*Mentha x piperita*) leaf
- ROSE (*Rosa* spp.) petal
- ROSEMARY (*Salvia rosmarinus*) leaf
- SPEARMINT (*Mentha spicata*) leaf
- STAR ANISE (*Illicium verum*) seed pod
- STEVIA (*Stevia rebaudiana*) leaf
- TULSI (*Ocimum tenuiflorum*) aerial parts
- VANILLA (*Vanilla planifolia*) bean pod

*Aerial parts are the leaves and flowers of a plant, generally harvested from the top 6 inches of a plant

Incorporating Fruits

Fruit is another easy way to adjust the flavor of a tea blend. It can also give a tea blend a bit of color or texture if you think it's lacking, and thus can be a great way to improve its appearance, particularly if you'll be gifting the tea to someone.

Here are some common fruits that you can add to your tea blends.

COMMON FRUITS FOR TEAS

- APPLE
- BLACK CURRANT
- BLACKBERRY
- BLUEBERRY
- CRANBERRY
- GRAPE
- GRAPEFRUIT
- LEMON
- LIME
- MANGO
- ORANGE
- PEACH
- PEAR
- PINEAPPLE
- RASPBERRY
- STRAWBERRY

When adding fruit to a tea, you can use fresh or dried fruit. Fresh fruit is ideal for a single cup or pitcher of tea that will be drunk within 24-48 hours, whereas dried fruit is needed when you are creating a large batch of a tea blend that will be stored and used later.

When creating a large batch botanical tea blend (or adding fruit to one of your favorite tea blends in this book), the fruit must be thoroughly dried before adding it to the blend. You can purchase pre-dried fruit, or you can easily dry it yourself at home in the oven or dehydrator. To learn more about properly drying fruit for tea blends, check out our **Tea Blending 101 Mini Course**, where we share some tips on reducing moisture, maintaining flavor and color, and finding the proper temperature for drying.

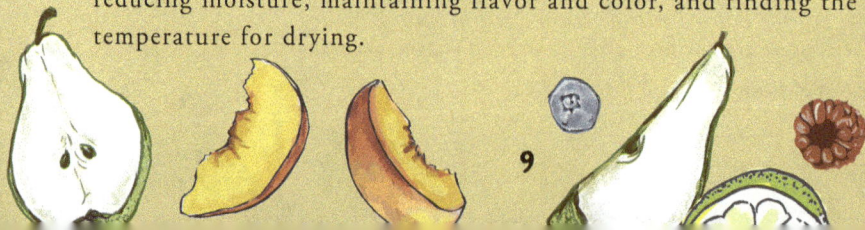

Incorporating Other Flavors *and* Aromas

An additional way to add taste and fragrance appeal to your tea blends is by incorporating GRAS (generally recognized as safe) essential oils, such as bergamot (*Citrus* x *bergamia*) peel, cinnamon (*Cinnamomum* spp.) leaf, and lemon (*Citrus* x *limon*) peel, into the dried blend. Adding essential oils is typically reserved for blends in which the desired flavor and aroma cannot be achieved using plant material alone. Very little essential oil is needed, and it's important to use a high quality essential oil.

While there are two recipes in this book that utilize essential oils, adding these preparations to tea blends is an advanced tea-making technique—one that is discussed in more depth in our **Tea Blending 101 Mini Course**—and must be approached with caution and thorough research.

Another way to incorporate additional flavor into a tea blend is by adding a smoke flavor to the blend if desired. You can do this by adding tea (*Camellia sinensis*) leaves that have already had a smoke flavor added to them, or you can use a food and drink smoke infuser to add the smoke flavor to the entire herbal tea blend. These are available online or in specialty tea shops.

Now that you know how to tweak the flavor and aroma of your botanical tea blends, let's look at the various methods of making herbal teas.

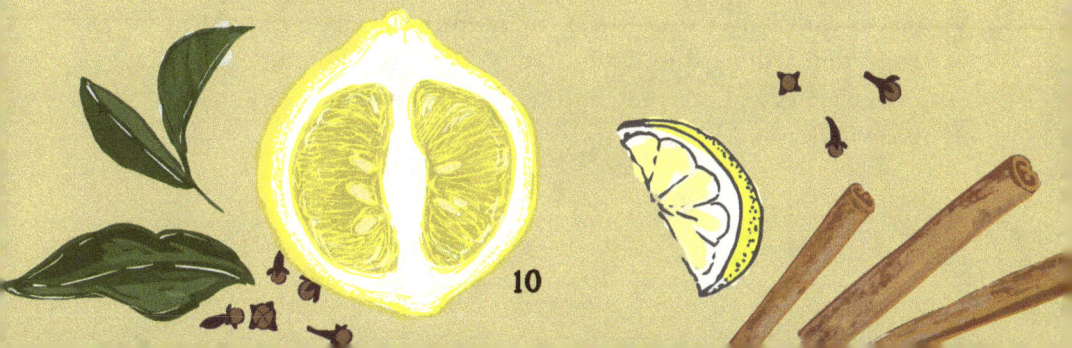

How To Make Herbal Tea

As we mentioned earlier, when it comes to extracting herbs in water, there are two main methods you need to know about—infusions and decoctions. These water extractions are generally quite simple to prepare, though there are some considerations to be aware of to ensure a well extracted beverage.

METHOD: What plant part are you working with? If you are working with a more delicate plant part, such as a flower or leaf, you will prepare your herbal tea as an infusion. If you are working with a hard plant part, such as a root, seed, or bark, then a decoction will be the way to go because the cell walls of these parts of the plant typically need higher heat and more time to extract their beneficial constituents.

SURFACE AREA: The size of the herb material impacts the efficiency of extraction. Imagine sticking a whole root into a jar and covering it with hot water. There will be some amount of extraction, but by breaking the root into smaller pieces, more of the plant's surface area will be exposed to the water. In general, the smaller the particle size, the more opportunity for constituent extraction. That does not mean that all herbs should be powdered; most often cut and sifted herbs (those that are processed into small pieces of uniform size) are perfect for herbal tea.

STEEP TIME: The recipes in this book include a suggested steep time for each individual blend. In general, the longer amount of time an herbal infusion is steeped, the more thorough the extraction. But that doesn't mean that steeping longer is always better! In the case of herbs rich in vitamins and minerals, a longer steep time is a good thing as it is needed to effectively extract those nutrients. On the other hand, herbs high in bitter or astringent constituents become more bitter and astringent with longer steep times, so in order to make a tasty blend the steep time will need to be shorter. We encourage you to experiment with steep times and take note of the changes to flavor, color, and extraction efficacy.

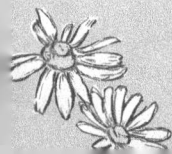

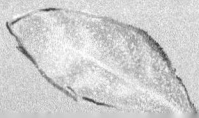

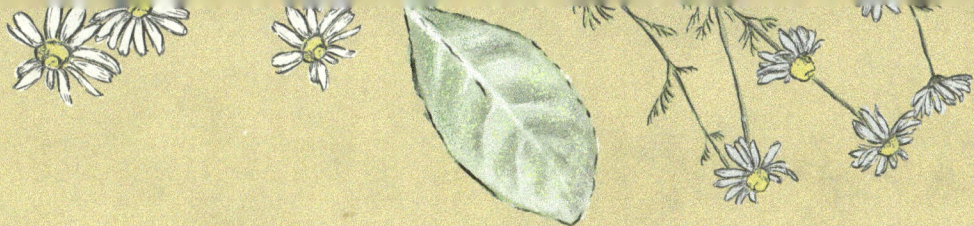

TEMPERATURE: Many herbal constituents are extracted more readily when heat is applied, as this heat bursts the cells walls of the plants, thus increasing extraction. However, sustained high temperatures, such as are used when making decoctions, can result in the breakdown of heat-sensitive constituents, such as some vitamins (e.g., vitamin C) and minerals. High temperatures can also cause the loss of volatile oils—for both infusions and decoctions, it is best to mitigate loss of aromatic compounds through volatilization during the heating process by covering with a lid during the extraction process.

In the case of mucilaginous plants such as marshmallow (*Althaea officinalis*) root and violet (*Viola* spp.) leaf and flower, cool water extraction is the most advantageous preparation, as heat breaks down the polysaccharides that are responsible for the slippery, cooling mucilage in these plants (that said, some mucilage is retained in a hot water extraction). Herbs high in volatile compounds also lend themselves well to cool water extraction, as the aromatic compounds are not lost due to heat.

HERB AMOUNT: In general, herbal teas geared toward flavor and enjoyment will use less herbal material, with a ratio of approximately 15 g (0.5 oz) herb per 1 quart (32 fl oz) water. Wellness blends intended to promote a physiological response for health benefits may use more herbal material for the same amount of water—approximately 30 g (1 oz) herb per 1 quart (32 fl oz) water for a leafy herb. However, these are simply rough guidelines, and there are no hard and fast rules when it comes to the ratio of herb to water when making herbal teas!

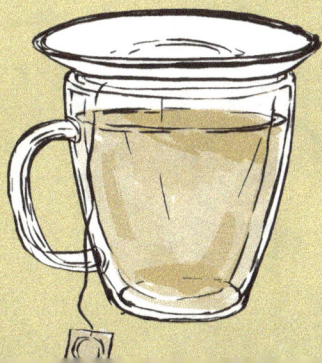

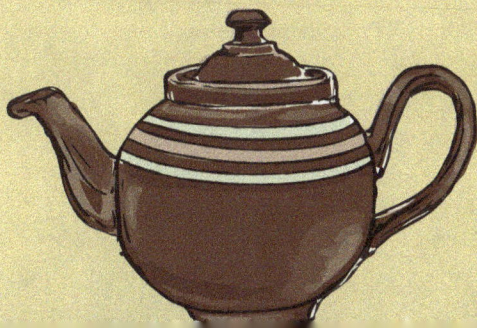

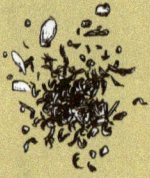
HERB
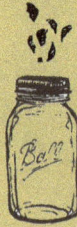
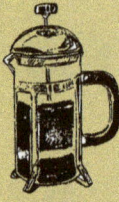
HEAT-SAFE CONTAINER
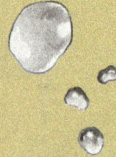
WATER
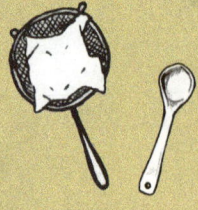
STRAINER

Preparing Tea

As previously mentioned, an herbal infusion is made by steeping herbs in water (this can be hot or cold water) and allowing the contact between the two to occur for the desired steep time. An herbal decoction is made by simmering plant parts and water in a pot on low heat for a sustained period of time, generally around 20 minutes. Here are general guidelines to follow when making teas using these methods.

HOT WATER INFUSIONS

1. Bring water to a boil in a kettle or pot.

2. While the water is heating, place herbs in a mug, heat-safe glass canning jar, French press, or teapot.

3. Pour hot water (wait until it stops boiling) over the herbs.

4. Cover the vessel to prevent volatile oils from escaping with the steam.

5. Steep for 5-20 minutes (or 4 hours to overnight, for a long-steeped infusion).

6. Filter the infusion using a tea strainer and a heat-safe vessel. Press down on the herbs with a spoon to squeeze out as much liquid as possible. If using a French press, just press and pour into your mug!

7. Consume immediately or within 24 hours after straining if refrigerated.

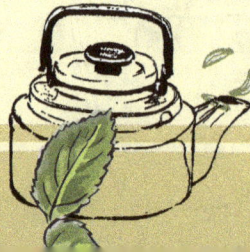

COLD WATER INFUSIONS

1. Place herbs in a mug, glass jar, French press, or teapot.

2. Pour room temperature or cool water over the herbs and cover.

3. Steep for 1 or more hours on the counter or in the refrigerator.

4. Filter the infusion using a tea strainer and a drinking vessel. Press down on the herbs with a spoon to squeeze out as much liquid as possible. If using a French press, just press and pour into your mug!

5. Consume immediately or within 24 hours after straining if refrigerated.

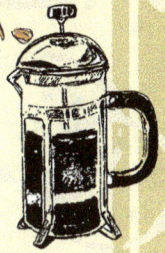

SOLAR INFUSIONS

Another option in herbal infusion making methodology is a solar extraction. This method utilizes the heat of the sun while steeping the water and herbs, creating a beautiful, sun-powered extraction. Most often you will start with cold or lukewarm water.

1. Place herbs and water in a glass jar, and cover tightly.

2. Place in a sunny spot for an hour or more (up to 8 hours).

3. Filter the infusion using a tea strainer and a drinking vessel. Press down on the herbs with a spoon to squeeze out as much liquid as possible.

4. Consume immediately or within 24 hours after straining if refrigerated.

NOTE: In any infusion prepared without high heat, there is a higher risk of potential bacterial growth. To minimize this, use clean equipment and filtered or boiled water, steep for just a couple hours, and store in the refrigerator.

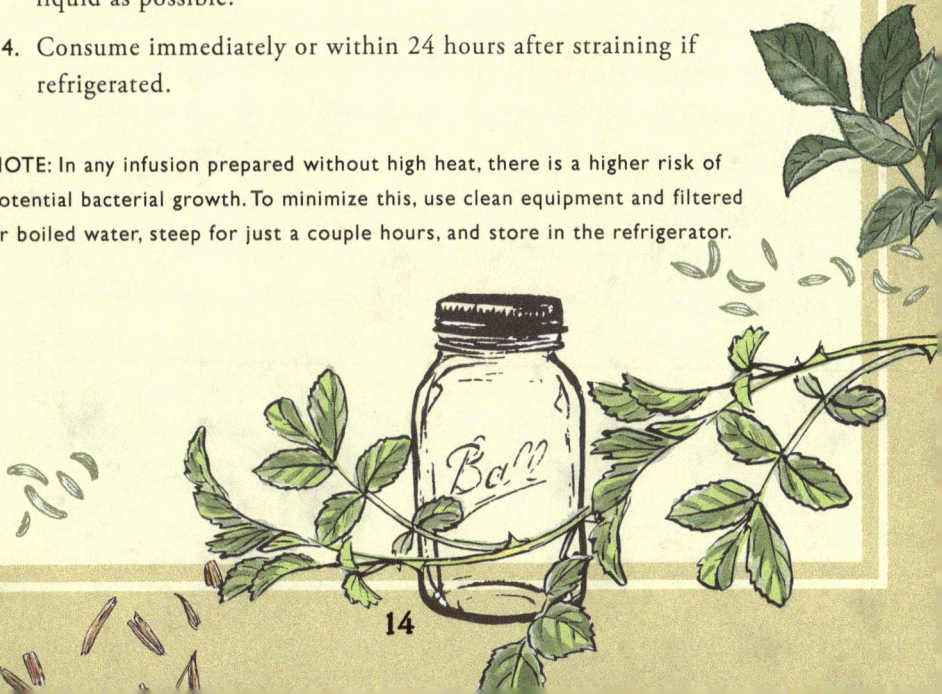

DECOCTIONS

To make a decoction, the water and herbs will be combined and simmered for a set period of time on a stovetop or other heat source. Remember, this method is most applicable to harder plant parts including roots, seeds, barks, and some berries.

1. Optional: soak herbs for a couple of hours or overnight prior to decocting to help soften the plant material.

2. Bring water and herbs to a boil in a covered pot, then lower the heat to a simmer.

3. Simmer for 20 minutes or more as directed in the recipe. Monitor the pot closely and turn down the heat if the water starts to boil.

4. Remove from heat and strain into a heat-safe vessel using a tea strainer.

5. Consume immediately or within 48 hours after straining if refrigerated.

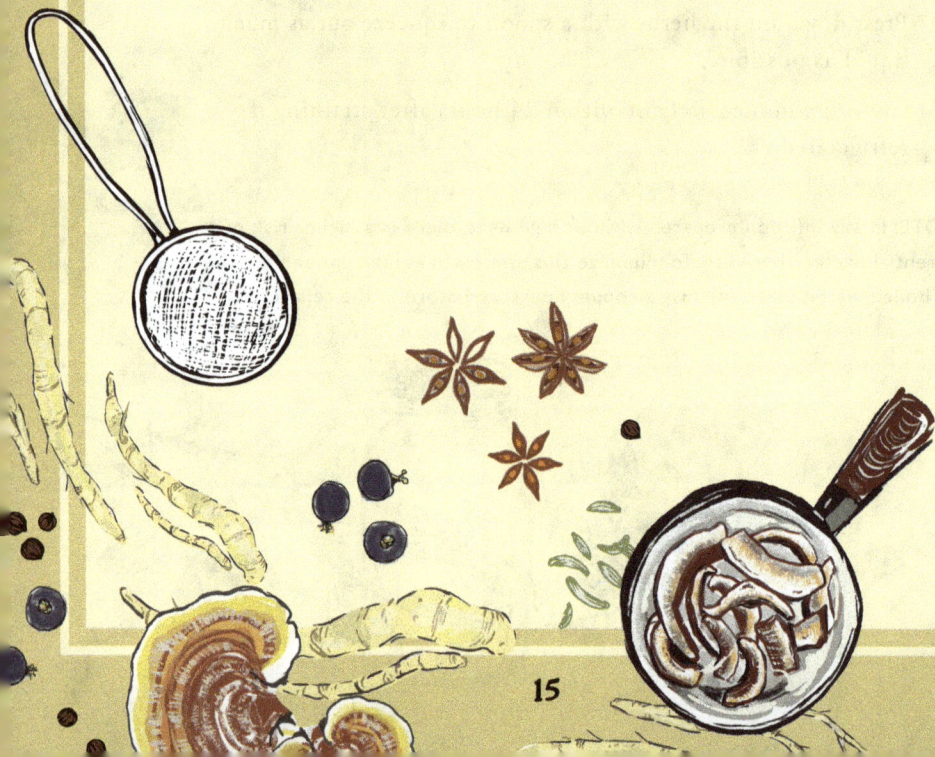

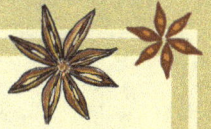

COMBINED INFUSION-DECOCTION

In some cases, depending on the plant parts included in a blend, it may be necessary to create both an infusion and a decoction to make the final product.

1. Decoct the roots/barks/seeds/fruits for a decoction.
2. Meanwhile, place leaves/flowers in a mug, heat-safe glass jar, French press, or teapot.
3. After 20 minutes or more of decocting, pour decocted herbs and hot water into the vessel with the leaves/flowers.
4. Cover and steep for 5-20 minutes (and up to 8 hours for a long-steeped infusion).
5. Filter the herb using a tea strainer and a heat-safe vessel. Press down on the herbs with a spoon to squeeze out as much liquid as possible. If using a French press, just press and pour into your mug!
6. Consume immediately or within 24 hours of straining if refrigerated.

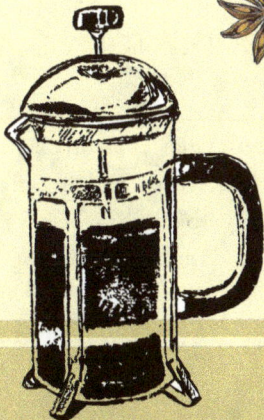

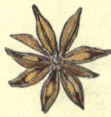

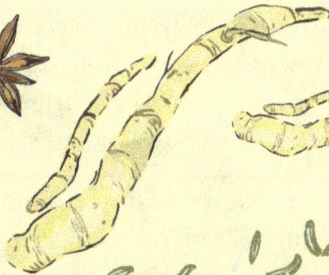

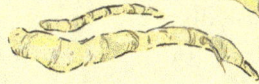

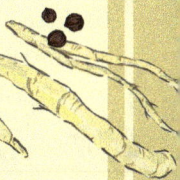

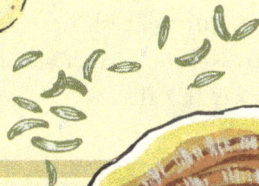

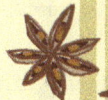

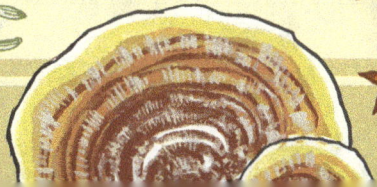

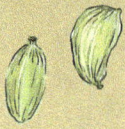

Storing *and* Reheating Prepared Tea

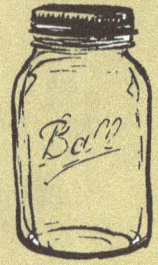

While many people make infusions and decoctions by the cup, you can certainly make a teapot or large canning jar full to prepare multiple servings at a time. While small batches of these water-based preparations are often consumed right away, it is a good idea to store larger amounts of an infusion or decoction in the refrigerator to minimize the chance of microbial growth. Infusions are stored for up to 24 hours in the refrigerator, whereas decoctions can be stored for up to 48 hours refrigerated before making a fresh batch.

When storing a leftover infusion or decoction in the refrigerator, you can enjoy the remainder of the preparation cold if you wish, or you can gently reheat it on the stove or in a kettle if you prefer to drink it warm. Keep in mind that reheating some herbal infusions or decoctions may lead to a bitter flavor, so you may want to add some extra flavorful herbs or sweetener in with the liquid when you reheat it if the taste becomes off-putting.

STORAGE AND SHELF LIFE OF TEA BLENDS

All herbs, fresh and dried, need to be stored in a cool, dark location to best preserve their properties.

Fresh herbs can be stored in the refrigerator. The aerial parts of fresh herbs (flowers and leaves) should ideally be used within 2-3 days as these will wilt relatively quickly (or they can be dried for later use). In contrast, harder parts of fresh herbs such as roots, barks, and berries will usually store for several weeks if refrigerated. Fresh herbs can also be placed in the freezer for up to 6 months.

When storing fresh herbs, it's vital to minimize oxygen exposure while keeping the plant moist. Fresh herbs do well when stored in bags that allow air to be pressed out, such as silicone storage bags, but beeswax wrap can also work. It's also a good idea to put a damp cloth or paper

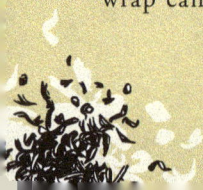

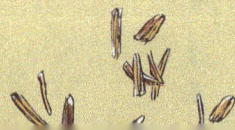

towel inside the bag with the herb to help maintain moisture and prevent the plant from drying out too quickly.

Some fresh herbs cannot be stored and must be used or dried as soon as they are harvested. Wild cherry (*Prunus serotina*) bark is one such herb. During the wilting process, the cyanogenic compound prunasin, found in wild cherry leaves and bark, hydrolyzes into the highly toxic hydrocyanic acid, which can be deadly in high amounts. This is why it is important to use either fresh or dried wild cherry leaf or bark. The same goes for red clover (*Trifolium pratense*) leaf and flowers—if not immediately prepared into a tincture or dried quickly and effectively, the coumarins in red clover can transform into a dangerous blood-thinning compound due to the development of mold. Therefore, it's essential to process or dry wild cherry bark and red clover flower immediately (and carefully!) to prevent fermentation or mold from developing. As with all herbs, it's vital to research any plant you are using so you are thoroughly aware of any safety precautions.

Dried herbs, on the other hand, are much easier to store. It's best to keep them in containers and locations that minimize exposure to oxygen, light, and moisture. Dried herbs can be stored in airtight glass jars or bags that can be placed in cabinets, on shelves, in closets, or even under your bed. The aerial parts of dried herbs (flowers and leaves) have a shelf life of around a year, whereas the harder parts of dried herbs (barks, roots, and berries) may stay potent for up to 2 years when stored properly.

Dried herbs can also be stored in the refrigerator or freezer, which will extend their shelf life slightly. For best practice, they should be packaged in small amounts in airtight containers. When you are ready to use an herb, either remove it from the refrigerator or freezer, use it quickly, and replace it before it comes to room temperature, or remove one smaller-sized package, leaving it stored in a cool, dark location in your home and using it completely before removing another from the refrigerator or freezer. The reason for this is that the temperature shift from cold to warm can allow moisture to come into contact with the dried plant material more easily, reducing its shelf life and increasing risk of spoilage.

Another factor that affects a plant's shelf life is its size. Plants processed into smaller pieces, such as chopped, shredded, or powdered herbs, will have a shorter shelf life than larger pieces or whole plant parts, as more of their surface is exposed to the elements. This is important to keep in mind when processing foraged herbs or choosing the form of an herb to purchase from a local herb shop or online supplier. When it comes to storing herbs for making tea blends, chances are you will be storing your herbs in dried form.

In the practice of tea making, there is deep nourishment that comes along with the plant allies. The simple act of extracting herbs into water can turn into a ritualistic experience if one so chooses. Practice mindful awareness and intention setting while working through the recipe steps provided for a fuller experience. And don't forget to sip, savor, and enjoy!

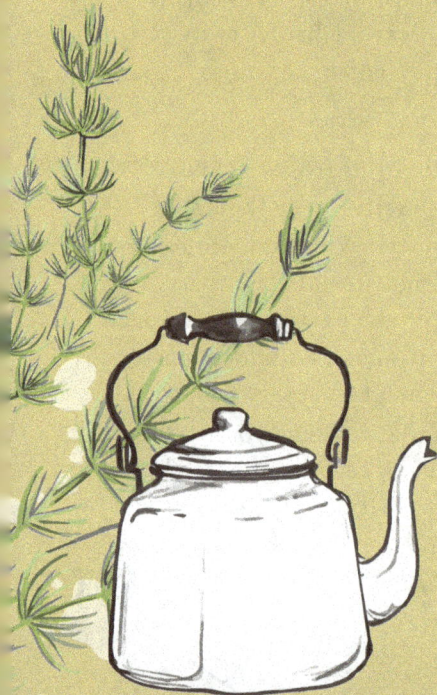

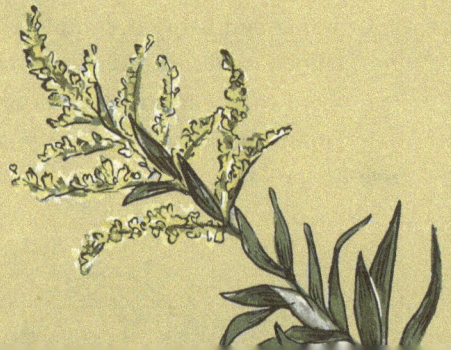

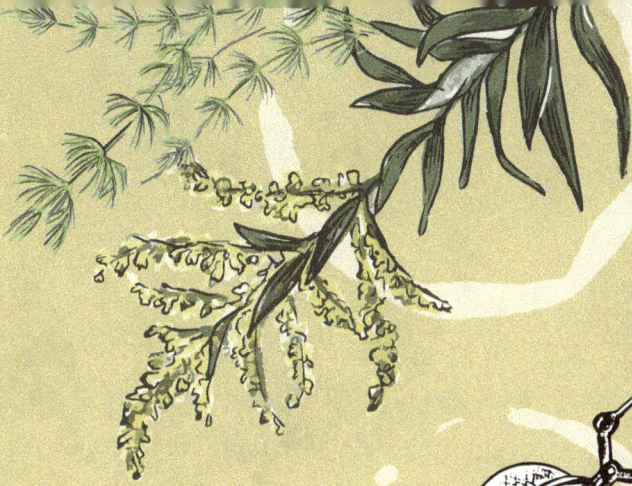

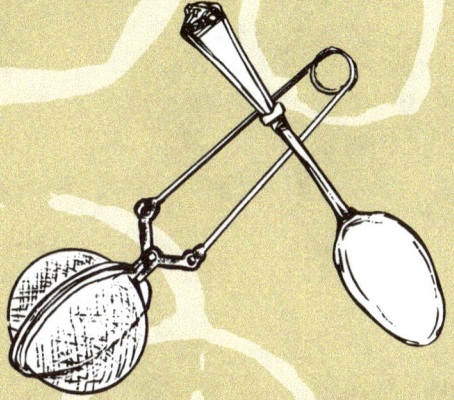

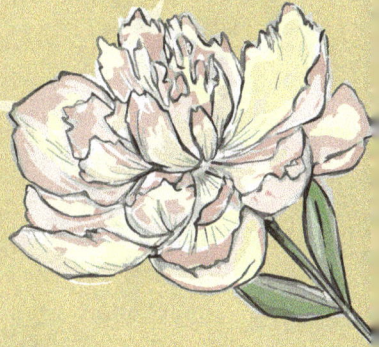

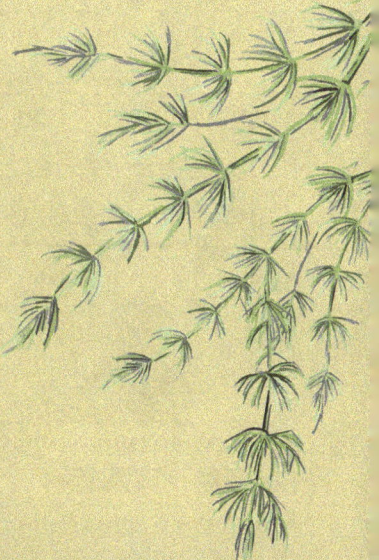

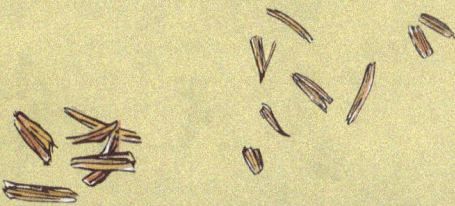

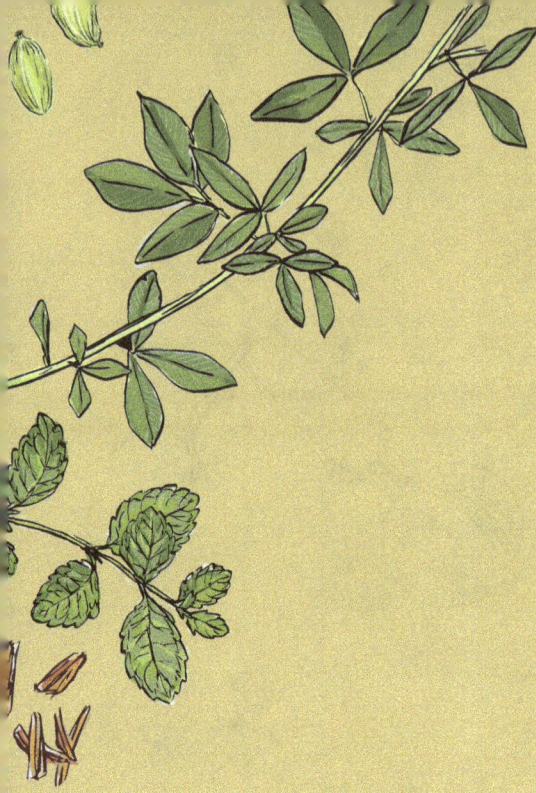

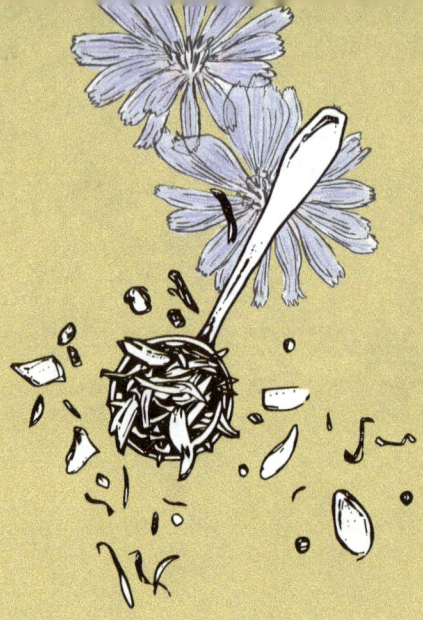

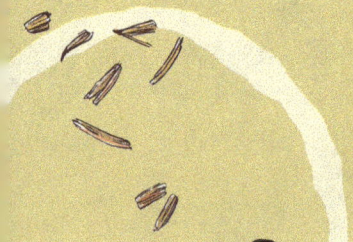

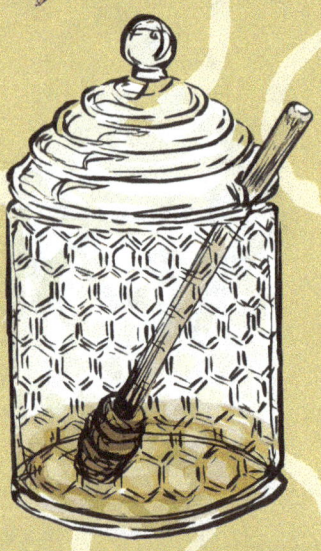

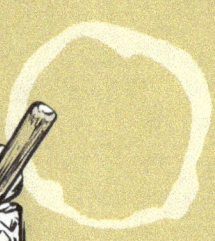

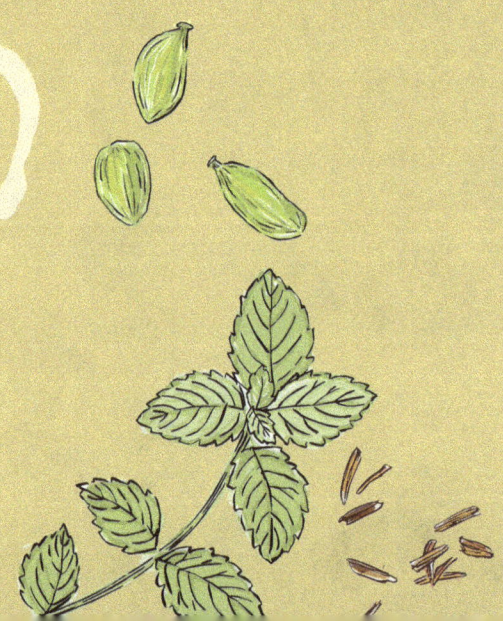

CHAPTER TWO
TEA NOTES

Here are some important notes to keep in mind as you craft dried botanical tea blends and brew the herbal teas in the recipes to follow in the next chapter.

Recipe Tips

All herb and fruit ingredients are dried unless otherwise noted as fresh. We suggest choosing organic, sustainably grown ingredients when possible.

Some tea blend recipes include powdered herbs, which may settle to the bottom of the container during storage. Give these blends a good mix to incorporate all herbs parts together before brewing so as to ensure that all herbs are distributed throughout the mixture.

Recipes that were formulated to include milk (dairy or non-dairy) and sweetener for maximum flavor and enjoyment list those in the ingredients list. Addition of milk or sweetener to other recipes is of course welcome based on your own personal preference.

- If a recipe calls for milk, feel free to use dairy milk or any non-dairy options you prefer, such as almond, coconut, or oat milk.

- Honey is a natural flavor pairing with herbal teas and has its own beneficial properties. If you prefer not to use honey, other sweetener options include maple syrup, herbal glycerites, or a pinch of stevia (*Stevia rebaudiana*) leaf.

As mentioned previously, if you have left over infusions or decoctions, those can be stored in the refrigerator and reheated or enjoyed cold or over ice. Infusions can be stored refrigerated for up to 24 hours, while decoctions can be stored refrigerated for up to 48 hours.

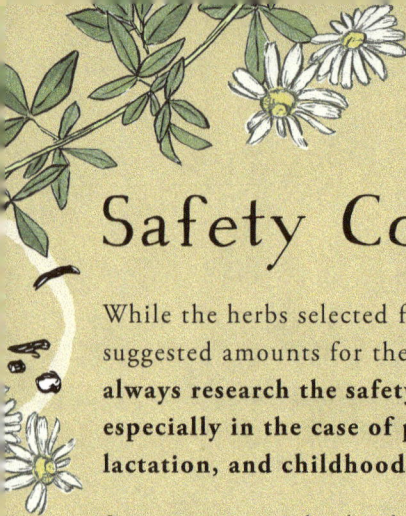

Safety Considerations

While the herbs selected for these recipes are typically safe in the suggested amounts for the general adult population, **it is important to always research the safety of individual herbs prior to consumption, especially in the case of particular health conditions, pregnancy, lactation, and childhood.**

Some recipes in this book include herbs that are widely used but also come with important safety considerations. Licorice (*Glycyrrhiza glabra*), which is commonly used in teas for flavor as well as its moistening mucilage and other beneficial actions, but should not be taken long-term (more than 6 weeks) or in high doses as it can cause an acute rise in blood pressure or edema. St. John's wort (*Hypericum perforatum*) interacts with a number of pharmaceutical drugs, particularly blood thinners and antidepressants by inducing CYP450 drug-metabolizing enzymes and a drug-transporter protein, and should generally be avoided while taking any pharmaceutical drug.

SPECIAL SAFETY CONSIDERATIONS: PREGNANCY

Both licorice and St. John's wort are also contraindicated in pregnancy and lactation, and of course there are many other herbs that should be avoided for those who are pregnant or nursing. While some herbs are considered safe in pregnancy, avoidance of any herb in the first trimester—even gentle tonic herbs like raspberry (*Rubus idaeus*) leaf—is recommended by some. **It's important to consult a health care provider as well as an experienced herbalist prior to consuming herbs during pregnancy.**

PREGNANCY FRIENDLY

This notation is used throughout the recipes in this book to denote formulations that are generally safe for use in moderate amounts during the second and third trimester of pregnancy and are considered safe when used in that way for the majority of pregnancies. However, every pregnancy is different, and it is

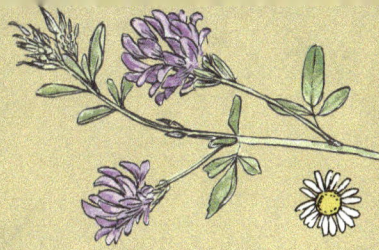

important to discuss all use of herbs with your health care provider prior to consuming them.

SPECIAL SAFETY CONSIDERATIONS: CHILDREN

While there are many kid-friendly herbs, children are another population for whom herb choices should be made conscientiously, with dosage adjusted for their body size. A simple method for doing this is to use Clark's Rule—divide a child's weight in pounds by 150 pounds (considered an average adult weight) to get the fraction of the adult dose that is appropriate for a child of that weight (e.g., for a 50-lb child, 50/150 = 0.3, so they would consume ⅓ of the adult dosage).

KID FRIENDLY

This notation is used throughout the recipes in this book to denote formulations that are generally kid-friendly for children ages 3 and up. These recipes include herbs that are generally thought to be safe for children in moderation and for short term use, however, each child is different and there is always the possibility of an idiosyncratic reaction or allergy. Serving sizes and dosage per day should be adjusted based on Clark's Rule as described above.

SPECIAL SAFETY CONSIDERATIONS: WILDCRAFTING

If foraging plants for use in these recipes, please follow foraging safety guidelines and ethics. Be 100% certain of the identification of a plant as well as its preparation requirements prior to using it in botanical teas.

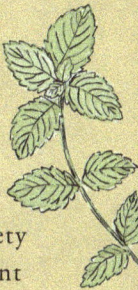

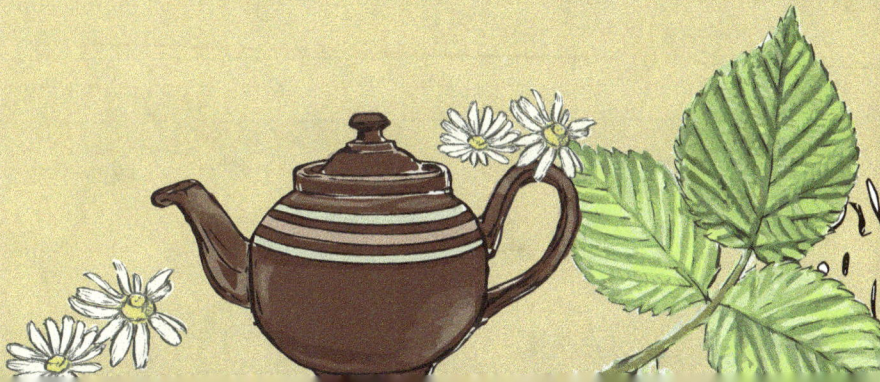

Recipe Notation Legend

KID FRIENDLY

Generally kid-friendly for children ages 3 and up in moderation and for short term use. Each child is different and there is always the possibility of an idiosyncratic reaction or allergy. Serving sizes and dosage per day should be adjusted based on Clark's Rule.

PREGNANCY FRIENDLY

Generally safe for use in moderate amounts during the second and third trimester of pregnancy and are considered safe when used in that way for the majority of pregnancies. Discuss all use of herbs with your health care provider prior to consuming them.

SHORT TERM USE

Short-term use of 2-4 weeks; these recipes should not be used by anyone long term.

NOTE: Please check in with an herbalist or healthcare provider if you plan to use any teas in this book long term. While they may be safe for some people used over a longer period of time, that is not the case for every person or health situation.

MEASUREMENT CONVERSION

I fl oz	2 tbsp	6 tsp	30 mL

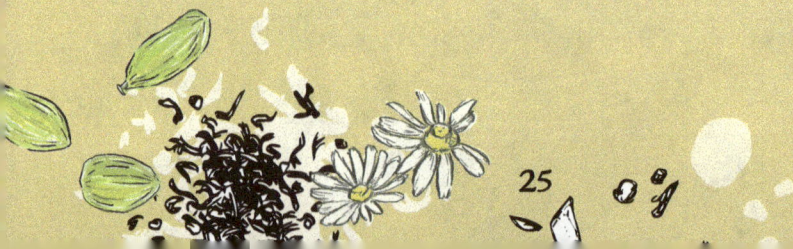

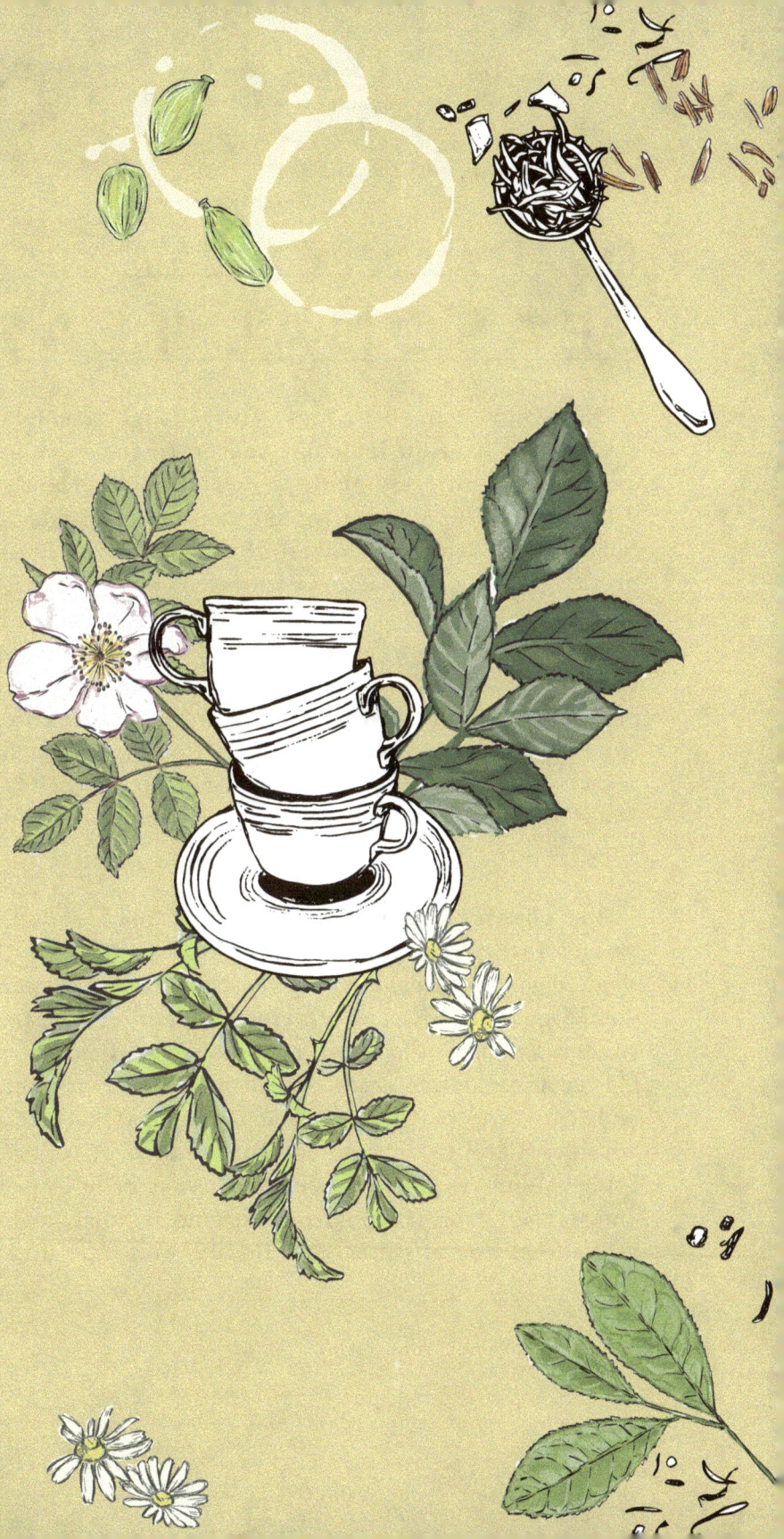

CHAPTER THREE
SEASONAL TEAS

As herbalists, our go-to teas often change throughout the year as we flow from one season to the next, and our bodies intuitively guide us toward the herbs that will provide the balance we are craving. This is a fundamental tendency for all of us, as we seek fresh greens in the spring after a winter of heavy foods, crisp, cool cucumbers in summer to offset the oppressive heat, or cozy, spiced stews in autumn and winter to warm us up. Of course there is a seasonality to the availability of produce and herbs that figures into our selections, but they are also heavily based on the energetics of the season—hot, cold, damp, dry—and our bodies' needs as we adapt to sweltering summer days or the chilly winds of autumn.

In this chapter, you will find botanical tea blends that reflect the seasons. An assortment of spring blends will awaken your senses, provide fresh nourishment, pep up your digestion, focus your attention, and celebrate the garden and the enlivening energy of this time of year. Our summer blends are all about bountiful fresh herbs and fruits and tasty ways to beat the heat with cooling botanicals and refreshing sun teas. The shift to autumn brings blends that celebrate the flavors of fall produce and warming spices, boost our immune systems, and dig into the power of roots. And finally, we settle into winter with herbal blends that keep us warm and cozy, provide deep nourishment and ongoing immune support, and cradle our hearts and minds with gentleness and calm that encourage the restorative rest that winter provides.

SECTIONS:

Spring

Botanical blends that will awaken your senses, provide fresh nourishment, pep up your digestion, focus your attention, and celebrate the garden and the enlivening energy of this time of year.

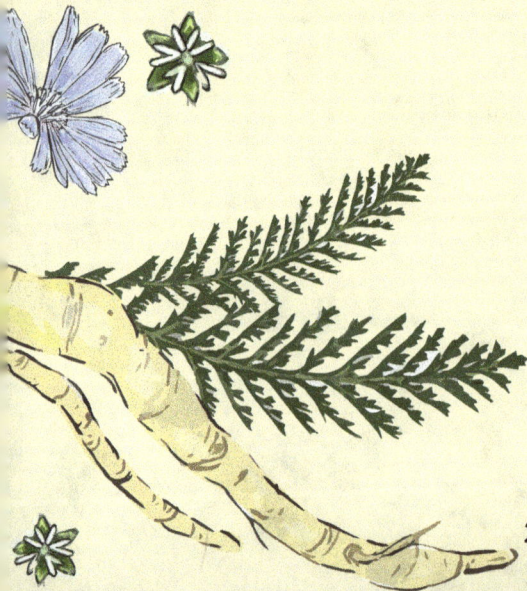

RECIPES:

Citrus Splash
MONDAY TEA

Start off the work week with this brain-boosting, citrus-full, made-for-Monday tea. Sure to get your mind moving after a weekend off, this tea not only tastes great but has the brain-boosting power of herbal allies to clear out the cobwebs for a fresh start! Feel free to substitute fresh peppermint or spearmint for the lemon balm.

Yield: Eight 8 fl oz servings

INGREDIENTS

1 fresh ruby red grapefruit, sliced

2 fresh lemons, sliced

½ cup fresh lemon balm (*Melissa officinalis*) aerial parts, chopped

¼ cup calendula (*Calendula officinalis*) flower

64 fl oz (1.9 L) water

Honey (or sweetener of choice) to taste (optional)

DIRECTIONS

Place all herbs and fruit ingredients in a heat-safe container.

Pour freshly boiled hot water over the herbs and fruit, cover, and steep for 15 minutes.

Strain the infusion through a tea strainer and compost or discard plant material.

Add honey, if desired.

Sip hot, or allow to cool and serve over ice.

Consume immediately or within 24 hours after straining, if refrigerated.

Drink up to eight servings per day.

| KID FRIENDLY

FULL MOON
floral tea

This tea is naturally tart, tangy, and pleasantly aromatic. Hibiscus calyxes impart a deep burgundy-cherry hue and rose petals add a heart-supportive floral effect. The combination of these two beautiful flowers benefits the skin, blood, nervous system, and physical and emotional heart. Brew a cup of this tea on a Full Moon night and soak in the moonlight as you sip.

Yield: 1½ cups dried tea blend

INGREDIENTS

1 cup hibiscus (*Hibiscus sabdariffa*) calyx

½ cup rose (*Rosa* spp.) petal

DIRECTIONS

Combine ingredients and store the blend in a labeled, tightly sealed storage container. Use within 12 months.

Steep 2 tbsp of tea blend per 8 fl oz (240 mL) freshly boiled hot water in a heat-safe container, covered, for 10-15 minutes.

Strain infusion through a tea strainer and compost or discard plant material.

Sip hot, or allow to cool and serve over ice, as you enjoy the flowering, full energy of the full moon and its emanating light.

Drink up to four 8 fl oz servings per day.

Garden Joy Blend

If you grow a garden, no matter the size, odds are you have mint tucked somewhere in there. Mint makes the perfect base for this garden blend, which follows no specific rules except for one: use what you have! Keep a large container of this blend on your apothecary shelf, and watch it continue to change as you continuously add to it throughout the seasons—sometimes more colorful, sometimes more minty, at times more orange, at others more blue. Let this blend be a reflection of your own garden and the edible flowers you have growing around you. Every time you head to the garden, collect a small quantity of edible flowers and mint leaves, feeling free to experiment with different mint family members, and allow the herbs to fully dry on a rack. Little by little, your garden joy blend will bulk up as you add dried flowers and leaves to the jar. This recipe is one example of what a cup of garden joy can taste like, but we'll let you take it from here!

Yield: One 8 fl oz serving

INGREDIENTS

2 tsp mint (*Mentha* spp.) leaf

1 tsp lemon balm (*Melissa officinalis*) aerial parts

1 tsp edible flowers of choice (single or as a mix), such as rose (*Rosa* spp.) petal, heartsease (*Viola tricolor*) flower, hollyhock (*Althaea rosea*) flower, calendula (*Calendula officinalis*) petal, etc.

8 fl oz (240 mL) water

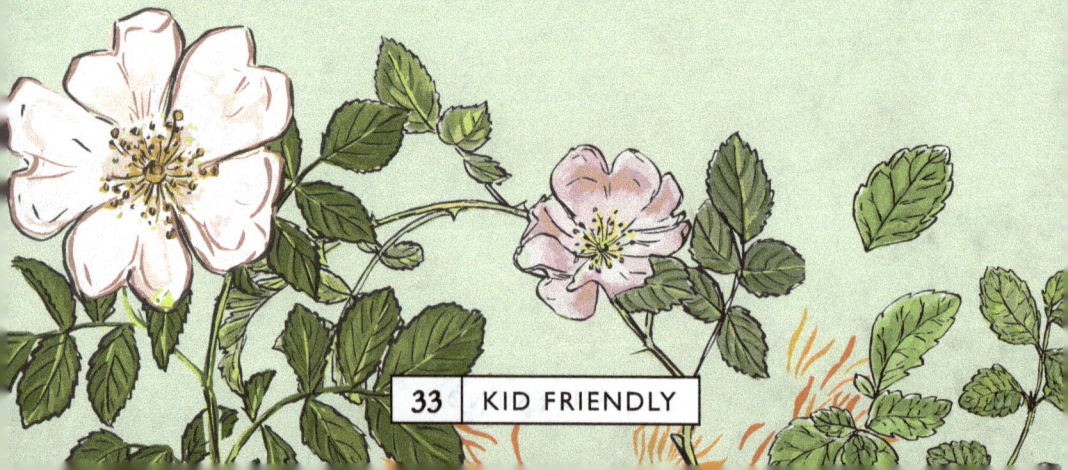

KID FRIENDLY

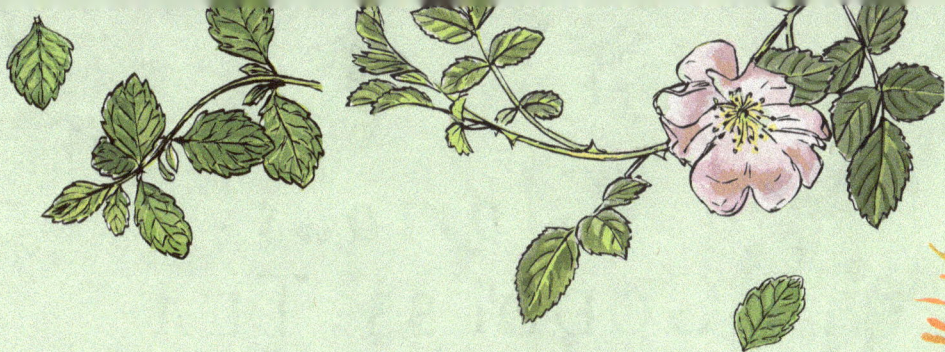

DIRECTIONS

Place herbs in a heat-safe container.

Pour freshly boiled hot water over the herbs, cover, and steep for 10-15 minutes.

Strain the infusion through a tea strainer and compost or discard plant material.

Serve and enjoy!

Drink up to four servings per day.

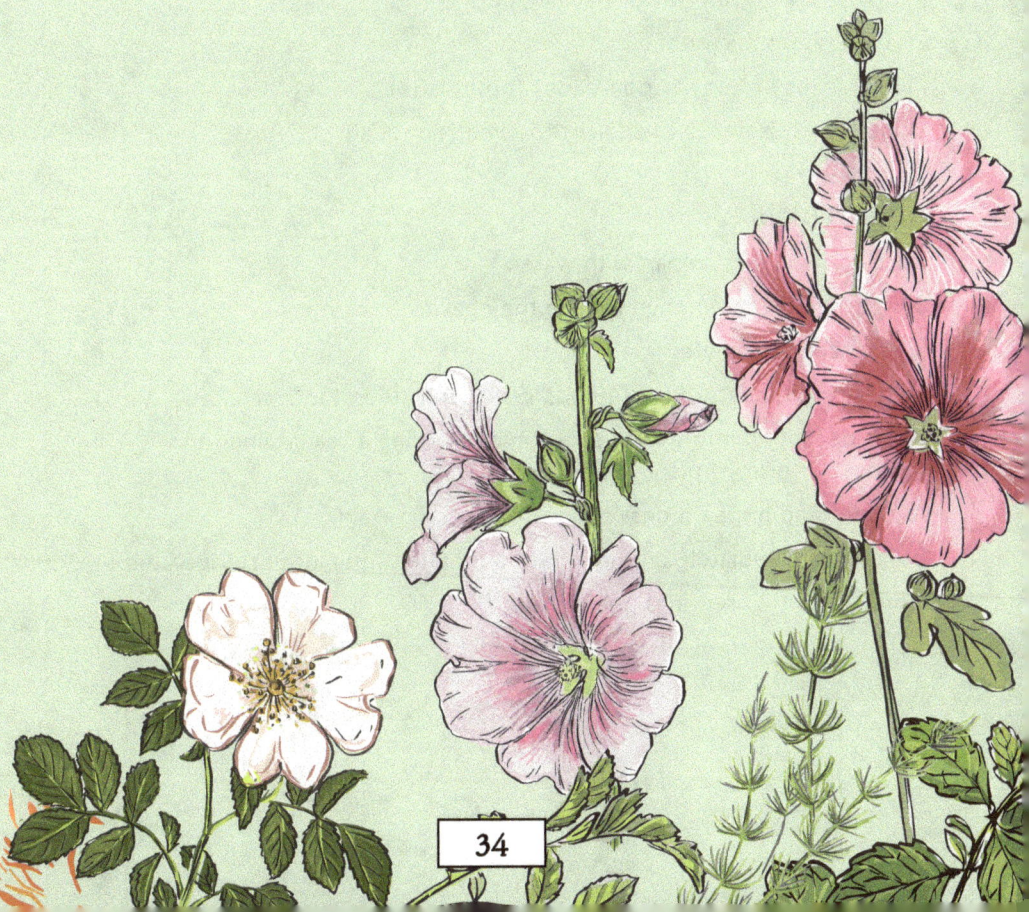

Glorious Goddess Tea

The pairing of these three herbs will help all who partake feel the divine in themselves. Shatavari, a member of the asparagus family, is renowned for its ability to empower through moisture and tone. This nourishing root is paired with white peony for its hormone-balancing effects, alongside rose to shine love inside yourself.

Yield: Approximately two 8 fl oz servings

INGREDIENTS

1 tbsp white peony (*Paeonia lactiflora*) root

1 tbsp shatavari (*Asparagus racemosus*) root

3-5 rose (*Rosa* spp.) flower buds or petals

24 fl oz (720 mL) water

Milk of choice (dairy or non-dairy) (optional)

Honey (or sweetener of choice) to taste (optional)

DIRECTIONS

Place roots in a saucepan with water.

Bring to a boil, cover, then reduce the heat to a simmer.

Simmer for 20 minutes.

Remove from heat, add rose buds, cover, and steep for 5 minutes.

Strain decoction into a heat-safe container using a tea strainer, and compost or discard plant material.

Add milk and honey, if desired.

Consume immediately or within 48 hours after straining, if refrigerated.

Drink up to two servings per day.

HERBAL ACADEMY'S
Nettle aLaLaLatte

If you're ready for nourishing spring herbs but still need some warming spices in your life, this recipe is just what you're looking for–perfect for those chilly spring mornings!

Yield: Approximately two 8 fl oz servings

INGREDIENTS

1 stick cinnamon (*Cinnamomum* spp.) bark, crushed

4 fresh ginger (*Zingiber officinale*) rhizome slices

1 tsp cardamom (*Elettaria cardamomum*) pods, crushed

½ tsp clove (*Syzygium aromaticum*) bud

24 fl oz (720 mL) water

2-4 tsp nettle (*Urtica dioica*) leaf

Milk of choice (dairy or non-dairy) to taste

Honey (or sweetener of choice) to taste

DIRECTIONS

Place all herbs except nettle in a saucepan with water.

Bring to a boil, cover, then reduce the heat to a simmer.

Simmer for 20 minutes.

Remove from heat, add nettle, cover, and steep for 30 minutes to overnight.

Reheat to drinking temperature, then strain decoction into a heat-safe container using a tea strainer, and compost or discard plant material.

Add milk and honey.

Consume immediately or within 48 hours after straining, if refrigerated.

Drink up to two servings per day.

| KID FRIENDLY

Raspberry Rose
"ICED" TEA

Iced tea is a summer staple that this recipe takes an herbal spin on, utilizing raspberry leaf and rose. These herbs not only taste great as an iced tea but they are also rich in nourishment and tonifying to the tissues. Give this a try on a hot summer day!

Yield: One 8 fl oz serving

INGREDIENTS

2 tsp raspberry (*Rubus idaeus*) leaf

1 tsp rose (*Rosa* spp.) petal

8 fl oz (240 mL) water

DIRECTIONS

Place herbs in a heat-safe mug or container.

Pour freshly boiled hot water over the herbs, cover, and steep for 10 minutes.

Strain the infusion through a tea strainer and compost or discard plant material.

Place in the refrigerator and allow to cool.

Serve over ice and enjoy!

Drink up to four servings per day.

'tis the Sneezin' tea

Are seasonal allergies keeping you inside? Enjoy the beautiful outdoors again after sipping this supportive tea blend!

Yield: 1½ cups dried tea blend

INGREDIENTS

½ cup nettle (*Urtica dioica*) leaf

½ cup goldenrod (*Solidago* spp.) aerial parts

¼ cup elder (*Sambucus nigra* or *S. canadensis*) flower

¼ cup yarrow (*Achillea millefolium*) aerial parts

DIRECTIONS

Combine all ingredients and store the blend in a labeled, tightly sealed storage container. Use within 12 months.

Steep 2 tsp of tea blend per 8 fl oz (240 mL) freshly boiled hot water in a heat-safe container, covered, for 10-15 minutes.

Strain the infusion through a tea strainer and compost or discard plant material.

Consume immediately or within 24 hours after straining, if refrigerated.

Drink up to four 8 fl oz servings per day.

Spring
DETOX BLEND

This spring detox blend includes herbs known to support liver function and provide essential nutrients for overall wellness.

Yield: Four 8 fl oz servings

INGREDIENTS

2 tsp dandelion (*Taraxacum officinale*) leaf

2 tsp nettle (*Urtica dioica*) leaf

2 tsp red clover (*Trifolium pratense*) aerial parts

2 tsp dandelion (*Taraxacum officinale*) root

2 tsp burdock (*Arctium lappa*) root

1 tsp lemon (*Citrus x limon*) or orange (*Citrus* spp.) peel

32 fl oz (960 mL) water

DIRECTIONS

Place herbs in a heat-safe container.

Pour freshly boiled hot water over the herbs, cover, and steep for 15 minutes.

Strain the infusion through a tea strainer and compost or discard plant material.

Consume immediately or within 24 hours after straining, if refrigerated.

Drink up to four servings per day.

Spring Greens Tea

During the spring season, we bask in the joy of the return of our green friends, saying hello once again to dandelion, chickweed, plantain, and more. It's no coincidence that these herbs are also wonderful detoxifying agents that get our lymph and blood moving after the more stagnant periods of the colder months. Enjoy this blend as you wake up the body from winter's slumber!

Yield: 2 cups dried tea blend

INGREDIENTS

½ cup dandelion (*Taraxacum officinale*) leaf

½ cup chickweed (*Stellaria media*) aboveground parts

½ cup violet (*Viola odorata* or *V. sororia*) leaf

¼ cup ground ivy (*Glechoma hederacea*) aboveground parts

¼ cup plantain (*Plantago* spp.) leaf

DIRECTIONS

Combine all ingredients and store the blend in a labeled, tightly sealed storage container. Use within 12 months.

Steep 2-3 tbsp of tea blend per 12 fl oz (360 mL) freshly boiled hot water in a heat-safe container, covered, for 10-15 minutes.

Strain infusion through a tea strainer and compost or discard plant material.

Drink up to four 12 fl oz servings per day.

Waxing Moon
HERBAL INFUSION

This calm and bright herbal infusion supports memory, healthy cognitive function, and a balanced nervous system all while soothing digestion. Peppermint lends a quality of brightness, gotu kola supports mental acuity, and lemon balm provides soothing upliftment. Since this blend is both relaxing and gladdening, it is appropriate to enjoy any day, or used ritually during the Waxing Moon.

Yield: 2¼ cups dried tea blend

INGREDIENTS

¾ cup gotu kola (*Centella asiatica*) leaf

¾ cup peppermint (*Mentha x piperita*) leaf

¾ cup lemon balm (*Melissa officinalis*) aerial parts

DIRECTIONS

Combine all ingredients and store the blend in a labeled, tightly sealed storage container. Use within 12 months.

Steep 2 tbsp of tea blend per 8 fl oz (240 mL) freshly boiled hot water in a heat-safe container, covered, for 10-15 minutes.

Strain infusion through a tea strainer and compost or discard plant material.

Sip hot, or allow to cool and serve over ice, as you enjoy the energy of the waxing moon.

Drink up to four 8 fl oz servings per day.

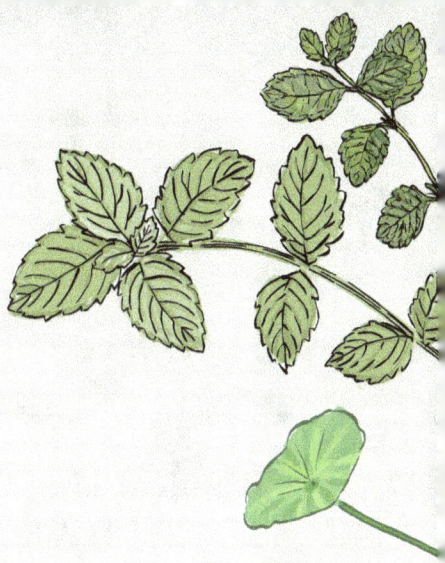

When creating your own herbal tea blends, one of the most important things you can do is spend time playing around in your kitchen and taking good notes on flavorful herbal combinations that you enjoy.

HERBAL ACADEMY'S
TEA BLENDING 101 MINI COURSE

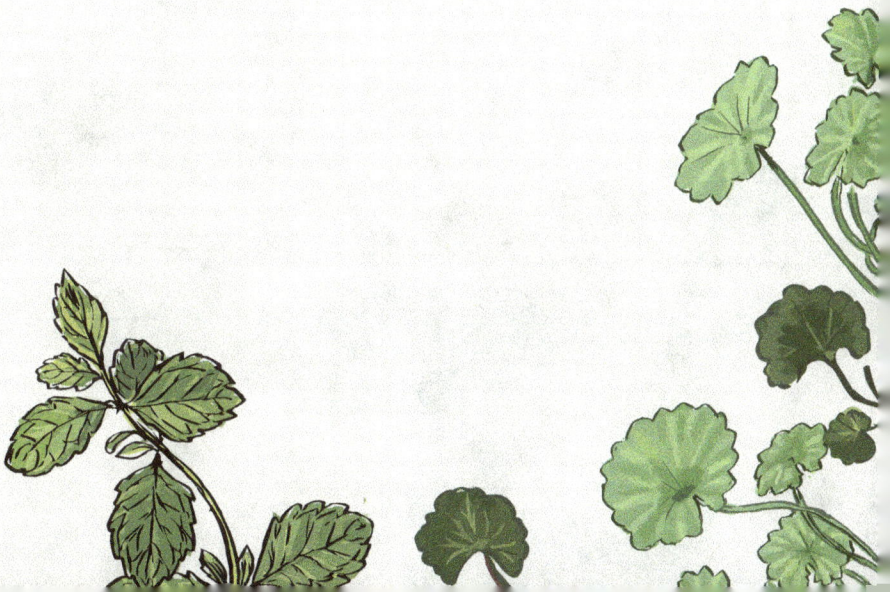

Summer

Botanical blends that bring together bountiful fresh herbs and fruits and tasty ways to beat the heat with cooling botanicals and refreshing sun teas.

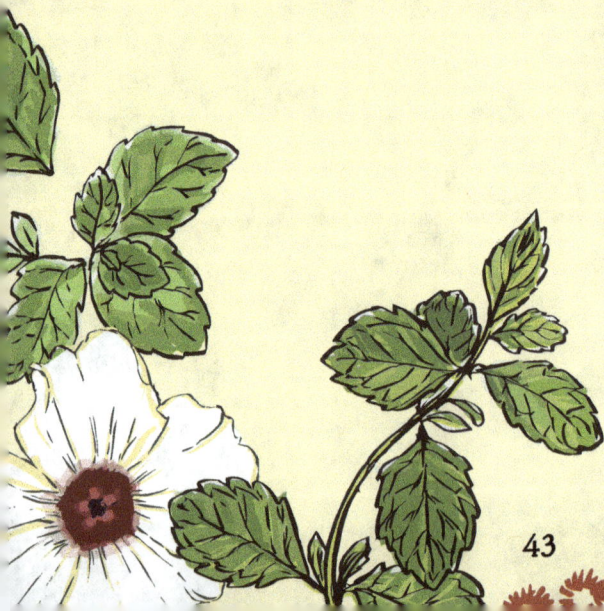

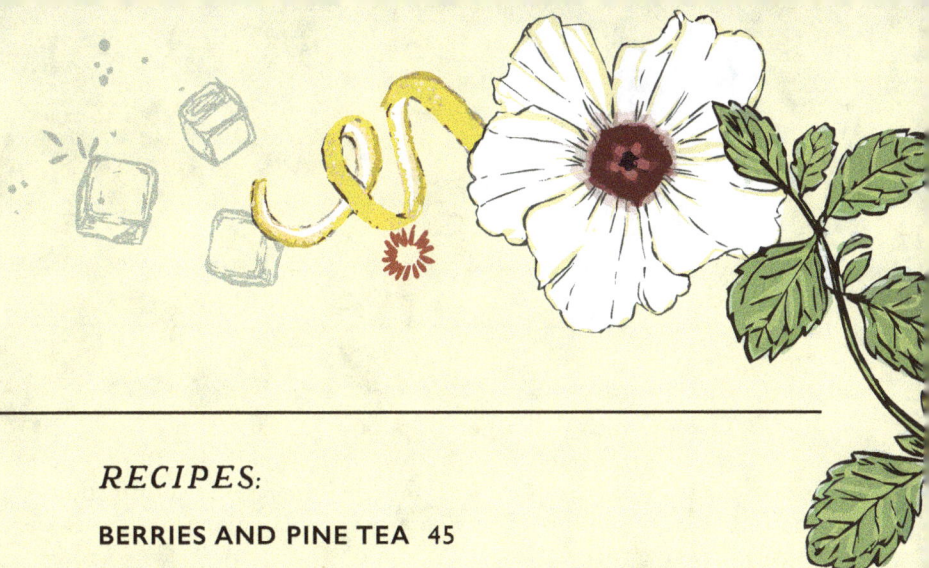

RECIPES:

Berries & Pine Tea

Both visually beautiful and potently flavorful, this recipe is a treat! The tart fruit profiles of lime and blueberries, paired with pine and lavender, create a zesty combination sure to please. If you so choose, add in butterfly pea flowers for an extra pop of color from the abundant polyphenol content.

Yield: Eight 8 fl oz servings

INGREDIENTS

½ cup fresh blueberries

¼ cup fresh lime, sliced

¼ cup fresh pine (*Pinus* spp.) needle, chopped

1 tbsp lavender (*Lavandula* spp.) flower bud (or fresh sprigs if you have some)

½ tsp fresh orange zest

1 pinch butterfly pea (*Clitoria ternatea*) flower for extra color (optional)

64 fl oz (1.9 L) water

DIRECTIONS

Place herbs and fruit ingredients in a heat-safe container.

Pour freshly boiled hot water over the herbs and fruit, cover, and steep for 15 minutes.

Strain the infusion through a tea strainer and compost or discard plant material.

Sip hot, or allow to cool and serve over ice.

Consume immediately or within 24 hours after straining, if refrigerated.

Drink up to four servings per day.

Cooling
ALLIES TEA

A blend of energetically cooling and moistening herbs to help beat the heat on a hot summer's day or soothe hot, inflamed tissues.

Yield: Two 8 fl oz servings

INGREDIENTS

2 tsp marshmallow (*Althaea officinalis*) root

2 tsp violet (*Viola odorata* or *V. sororia*) aerial parts

2 tsp linden (*Tilia* spp.) flower and bract

16 fl oz (480 mL) water

DIRECTIONS

Place herbs in a heat-safe container.

Pour freshly boiled hot water over the herbs, cover, and steep for 10-15 minutes.

Strain the infusion through a tea strainer and compost or discard plant material.

Serve and enjoy!

Consume immediately or within 24 hours after straining, if refrigerated.

Drink up to four servings per day.

COOL OFF
Minty Sun Tea

A wonderfully cooling pick-me-up for a hot summer's day. Peppermint is the perfect herb to help beat the heat, as its phytochemical constituent menthol acts on our thermoregulatory receptors in a way that tricks our body into believing it is cooled!

Yield: Eight 8 fl oz servings

INGREDIENTS

½ cup fresh peppermint (*Mentha x piperita*) leaf

½ cup fresh lemon balm (*Melissa officinalis*) aerial parts

½ cup fresh orange or lemon slices

64 fl oz (1.9 L) water

DIRECTIONS

Place herbs and fruit ingredients in a glass jar, and cover tightly.

Place in a sunny spot for 2-3 hours.

Strain the infusion through a tea strainer and compost or discard plant material.

Consume immediately or within 24 hours after straining, if refrigerated.

Drink up to eight servings per day; up to four servings per day if pregnant.

NOTES

In any infusion prepared without high heat, there is a higher risk of potential bacterial growth. To minimize this, use clean equipment, filtered or boiled water, steep in the sun for just a couple hours, and store in the refrigerator.

Easy Does It
SUN TEA

Drink a cup of sunshine tea under the sun as an exciting way to start off the summer season, and feel the calmness wash over you with each sip.

Yield: Four 8 fl oz servings

INGREDIENTS

2 tbsp linden (*Tilia* spp.) flower and bract

1 tbsp calendula (*Calendula officinalis*) flower

3 fresh lemon slices

32 fl oz (960 mL) water

DIRECTIONS

Place herbs and fruit ingredients in a glass jar, and cover tightly.

Place in a sunny spot for 2-3 hours.

Strain the infusion through a tea strainer and compost or discard plant material.

Consume immediately or within 24 hours after straining, if refrigerated.

Drink up to four servings per day.

NOTES

In any infusion prepared without high heat, there is a higher risk of potential bacterial growth. To minimize this, use clean equipment, filtered or boiled water, steep in the sun for just a couple hours, and store in the refrigerator.

| KID FRIENDLY

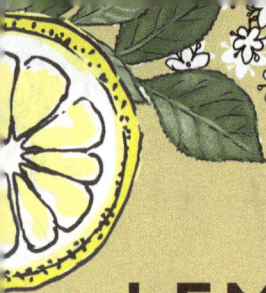
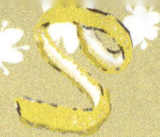

Elderflower
LEMON BALM "ADE"

An herbal take on lemonade, this recipe utilizes lemon balm to impart that lemony flavor. Paired with elderflower for a floral twist the end result is a cooling, refreshing tea best served over ice and sweetened with honey.

Yield: One 8 fl oz serving

INGREDIENTS

2 tsp elder (*Sambucus nigra* or *S. canadensis*) flower

1 tsp lemon balm (*Melissa officinalis*) aerial parts

8 fl oz (240 mL) water

1 tbsp (15 mL) lemon juice, freshly squeezed

Honey (or sweetener of choice) to taste

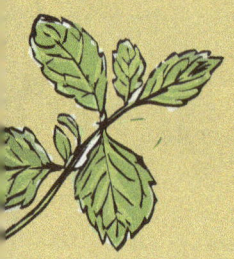
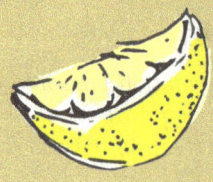
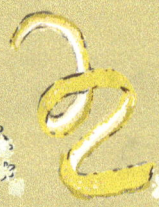
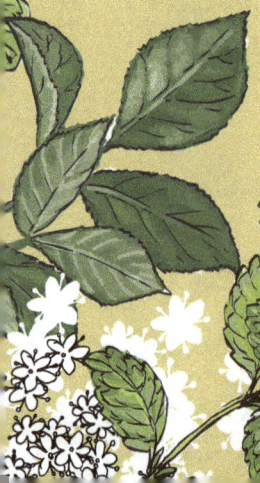
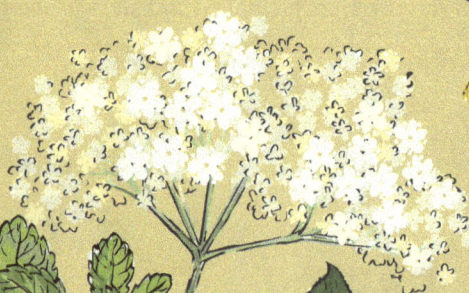
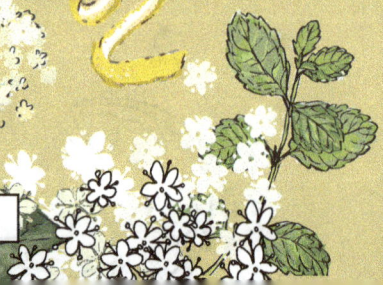

49 | KID FRIENDLY

DIRECTIONS

Place herbs in a heat-safe mug or container.

Pour freshly boiled hot water over the herbs, cover, and steep for 10-15 minutes.

Strain the infusion through a tea strainer and compost or discard plant material.

Sweeten with honey.

Place in the refrigerator and allow to cool.

Serve over ice and enjoy!

Drink up to four servings per day.

ELDERFLOWER
Vanilla Rooibos Delight

Calling all rooibos fans! This classic pairing of rooibos and vanilla is sure to delight the palates of many tea drinkers. This not-to-be-missed blend takes on a fun and unique twist with the addition of elderflower and toasted coconut, creating a unique and flavorful herbal combination.

Yield: One 8 fl oz serving

INGREDIENTS

1 tsp red rooibos (*Aspalathus linearis*) leaf

1 tsp elder (*Sambucus nigra* or *S. canadensis*) flower

1 tsp coconut flakes, toasted

8 fl oz (240 mL) water

½ tsp (2.5 mL) vanilla (*Vanilla planifolia*) extract

Honey (or sweetener of choice) to taste (optional)

DIRECTIONS

Place herbs and coconut flakes in a heat-safe mug or container.

Pour freshly boiled hot water over the herbs, cover, and steep for 10 minutes.

Strain the infusion through a tea strainer and compost or discard plant material.

Add vanilla extract and honey, if desired.

Sip and enjoy!

Drink up to four servings per day.

HERBAL ACADEMY'S
Summer Days Iced Tea

This perfectly pink tea packs a tart punch that is just the thing you need on a hot summer day in the sun. Not only will it help cool you down, but it is also loaded with vitamin C so you can stay energized and healthy all summer long!

Yield: 1⅜ cups dried tea blend

INGREDIENTS

½ cup violet (*Viola odorata* or *V. sororia*) leaf

½ cup lemon balm (*Melissa officinalis*) aerial parts

¼ cup hibiscus (*Hibiscus sabdariffa*) calyx

2 tbsp rose (*Rosa* spp.) hip

DIRECTIONS

Combine all ingredients and store the blend in a labeled, tightly sealed storage container. Use within 12 months.

Steep 1 tbsp of tea blend per 8 fl oz (240 mL) freshly boiled hot water in a heat-safe container, covered, for 20-30 minutes.

Strain infusion through a tea strainer and compost or discard plant material.

Place in the refrigerator and allow to cool.

Serve over ice with fresh sliced lemon round and enjoy!

Drink up to four 8 fl oz servings per day.

KID FRIENDLY

Herbal Paradise
SUN PUNCH

Pour this sun tea over ice with a little honey for sweetness, and you'll have an herbal paradise punch, perfect for sipping in the sunshine!

Yield: Four 8 fl oz servings

INGREDIENTS

2 tbsp hibiscus (*Hibiscus sabdariffa*) calyx

1 tbsp rose (*Rosa* spp.) hip

1 tbsp cinnamon (*Cinnamomum* spp.) bark, crushed

3 fresh orange slices

32 fl oz (960 mL) water

DIRECTIONS

Place all ingredients in a glass jar, and cover tightly.

Place in a sunny spot for 2-3 hours.

Strain the infusion through a tea strainer and compost or discard plant material.

Consume immediately or within 24 hours after straining, if refrigerated.

Drink up to four servings per day.

NOTES

In any infusion prepared without high heat, there is a higher risk of potential bacterial growth. To minimize this, use clean equipment, filtered or boiled water, steep in the sun for just a couple hours, and store in the refrigerator.

HIBISCUS
herbal cooler

Cool off with a cup of this rosy red blend that encourages release of body heat to reduce uncomfortable heat symptoms on a hot summer's day. Once your temperature starts to lower, you'll also start to unwind and notice that overactive mind start to relax thanks to some of our favorite nervines, chamomile and rose.

Yield: Eight 8 fl oz servings

INGREDIENTS

¼ cup hibiscus (*Hibiscus sabdariffa*) calyx

¼ cup chamomile (*Matricaria chamomilla*) flower

2 tbsp rose (*Rosa* spp.) hip

1 tbsp cinnamon (*Cinnamomum* spp.) bark, crushed

64 fl oz (1.9 L) water

Honey (or sweetener of choice) to taste

DIRECTIONS

Place herbs in a heat-safe container.

Pour freshly boiled hot water over the herbs, cover, and steep for 30 minutes.

Strain the infusion through a tea strainer and compost or discard plant material.

Sweeten with honey (or sweetener of choice) to taste, if desired.

Place in the refrigerator and allow to cool.

Serve over ice and enjoy!

Consume immediately or within 24 hours after straining, if refrigerated.

Drink up to eight servings per day.

Oh So Cool
PITTA POWER-DOWN TEA

Keep cool with this herbal tea blend for midday. Aimed at balancing *pitta dosha*, this combination soothes the nerves and gently stimulates digestion while easing imbalances, such as reflux and indigestion. Since 10 AM to 2 PM is considered the time of day in which *pitta dosha* is most prominent, if you find yourself feeling fiery, overly focused, or agitated at that time, try a cup of this cooling herbal tea blend.

Yield: Approximately four 8 fl oz servings

INGREDIENTS

2 tbsp marshmallow (*Althaea officinalis*) root

1 tbsp spearmint (*Mentha spicata*) leaf

1 tbsp chamomile (*Matricaria chamomilla*) flower

1 tbsp hibiscus (*Hibiscus sabdariffa*) calyx

1 tbsp coriander (*Coriandrum sativum*) seed

1 tbsp cinnamon (*Cinnamomum* spp.) bark, crushed

1 tbsp fennel (*Foeniculum vulgare*) seed

½ tsp rose (*Rosa* spp.) petal

3-4 cardamom (*Elettaria cardamomum*) pods, crushed

32 fl oz (960 mL) water

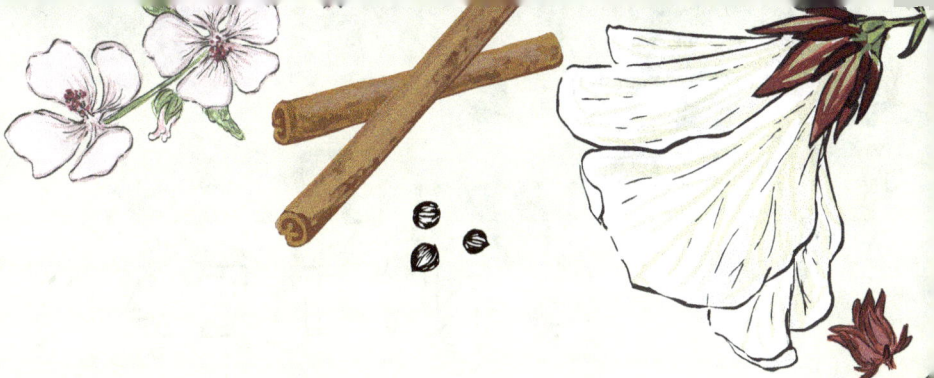

DIRECTIONS

Place roots, bark, seeds, and pods in a saucepan with water.

Bring to a boil, cover, then reduce the heat to a simmer.

Simmer for 5 minutes.

Remove from heat, add remaining herbs, cover, and steep for 5 minutes.

Strain decoction into a heat-safe container using a tea strainer, and compost or discard plant material.

Consume immediately or within 48 hours after straining, if refrigerated.

Drink up to four servings per day.

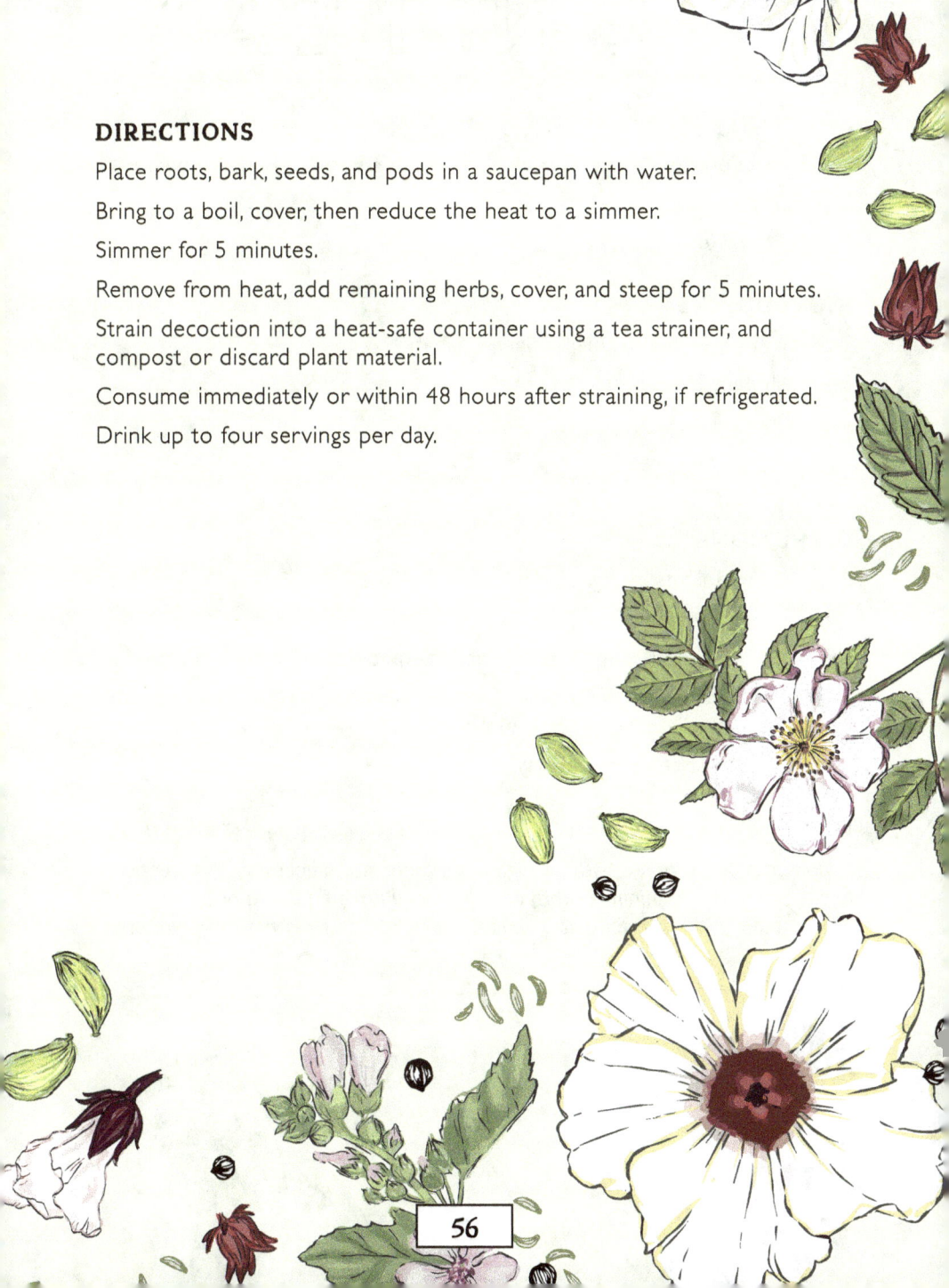

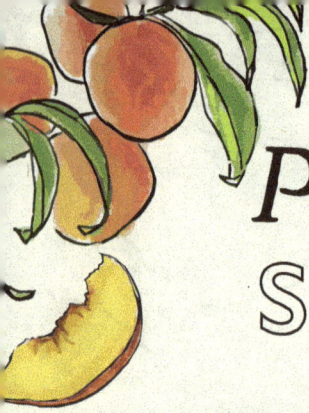

Peppy Peach
SUN TEA

With peaches in season, this peppy tea is perfectly timed for summer. We don't know about you, but we find that a summer peach is always refreshing!

Yield: Four 8 fl oz servings

INGREDIENTS

2 tea bags green tea (*Camellia sinensis*) leaf

3-5 fresh mint (*Mentha* spp.) sprigs

3 fresh peach slices

32 fl oz (960 mL) water

DIRECTIONS

Place all ingredients in a glass jar, and cover tightly.

Place in a sunny spot for 2-3 hours.

Strain the infusion through a tea strainer and compost or discard plant material.

Consume immediately or within 24 hours after straining, if refrigerated.

Drink up to four servings per day.

NOTES

In any infusion prepared without high heat, there is a higher risk of potential bacterial growth. To minimize this, use clean equipment, filtered or boiled water, steep in the sun for just a couple hours, and store in the refrigerator.

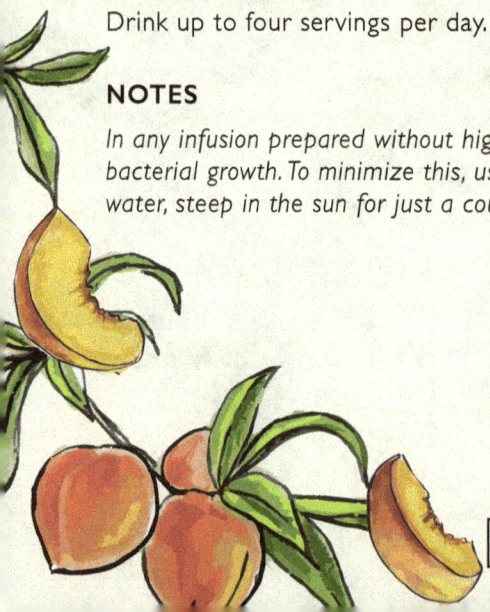

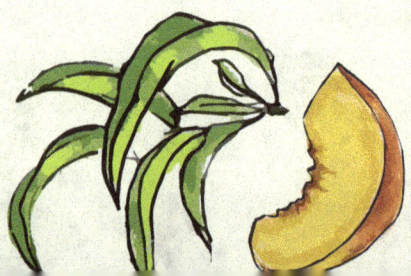

SOLAR SPLASH
sun tea

This nutritive blend of herbs will make a colorful and tasty batch of sun tea. Solar infusions will effectively extract the nutrients and the flavors alike! Perfect for a cooling cup after a long day outdoors in the summer sun.

Yield: 1⅝ cups dried tea blend

INGREDIENTS

½ cup sumac (*Rhus* spp.) berry

½ cup raspberry (*Rubus idaeus*) leaf

¼ cup hibiscus (*Hibiscus sabdariffa*) calyx

¼ cup blood orange (*Citrus* spp.) fruit

2 tbsp stevia (*Stevia rebaudiana*) leaf

DIRECTIONS

Combine all ingredients and store the blend in a labeled, tightly sealed storage container. Use within 12 months.

Steep ½ cup of tea blend per 32 fl oz (960 mL) water in a glass jar, and cover tightly.

Place in a sunny spot for 2-3 hours.

Strain the infusion through a tea strainer and compost or discard plant material.

Add honey (or sweetener of choice) to taste, and serve over ice.

Consume immediately or within 24 hours after straining, if refrigerated.

Drink up to four 8 fl oz servings per day.

NOTES

In any infusion prepared without high heat, there is a higher risk of potential bacterial growth. To minimize this, use clean equipment, filtered or boiled water, steep in the sun for just a couple hours, and store in the refrigerator.

Strawberry Basil
INFUSION

A classic flavor combo of strawberry and basil tastes like a warm summer day. This blend is sure to entice the senses, while cooling the mind and the body.

Yield: Four 8 fl oz servings

INGREDIENTS

1 fresh small cucumber, sliced
5 fresh large strawberries, sliced
6 fresh basil (*Ocimum basilicum*) leaves, sliced in thin strips
32 fl oz (960 mL) water

DIRECTIONS

Place all ingredients in a glass jar, and cover tightly.
Place in the refrigerator for 30 minutes.
Feel free to leave the ingredients in as you sip and enjoy!
Consume immediately or within 24 hours, if refrigerated.
Drink up to four servings per day.

SUMMER NIGHTS
Soothing After-Dinner Tea

This cooling blend of gentle carminatives is just the thing after a summer evening feast. Marshmallow root and coriander seed are well known for their soothing effects on heartburn and acid reflux—something you might experience more often in the summertime! Anise hyssop and blueberry round out the flavor while keeping the blend cooling and refreshing. Toasting coriander seeds is easy: simply heat a small pan on medium heat, add the untoasted seeds, and toast, stirring occasionally, until the aroma of coriander meets your nose.

Yield: Four 8 fl oz servings

INGREDIENTS

1 tbsp fresh or frozen blueberry fruit

1 tbsp coriander (*Coriandrum sativum*) seed, toasted

2 tsp marshmallow (*Althaea officinalis*) root

1 tsp anise hyssop (*Agastache foeniculum*) aerial parts

32 fl oz (960 mL) water

DIRECTIONS

Place herbs and fruit ingredients in a heat-safe container.

Pour freshly boiled hot water over the herbs, cover, and steep for 25-30 minutes.

Strain the infusion through a tea strainer and compost or discard plant material.

Serve and enjoy!

Consume immediately or within 24 hours after straining, if refrigerated.

Drink up to four servings per day.

turmeric
'ICED TEA' LEMONADE

This rich and refreshing turmeric lemonade tastes like sunshine on a warm day. A tasty beverage in its own right, but as a side hustle it works to reduce inflammation and ease pain (especially in the case of autoimmune conditions) due to its curcumin content, the polyphenol that not only adds color to this recipe but helps to downregulate inflammatory cytokines. This activity is further enhanced by a few pinches of black pepper, which increases curcumin's bioavailability.

Yield: Two 8 fl oz servings

INGREDIENTS

5 fresh mint (*Mentha* spp.) leaves (or basil (*Ocimum basilicum*) leaves), muddled

1 fresh lemon, freshly squeezed

2 tsp turmeric (*Curcuma longa*) rhizome, powdered

1 tsp (5 mL) maple syrup (or sweetener of choice) to taste

⅛ tsp black pepper (*Piper nigrum*) fruit, powdered

16 fl oz (480 mL) cold water

2 cups ice

1 sprig fresh mint (*Mentha* spp.), for garnish (optional)

1 fresh lemon wedge, for garnish (optional)

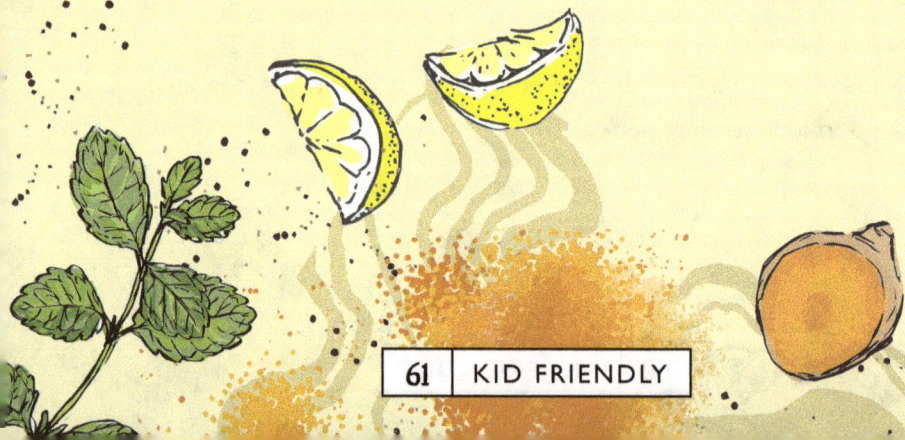

KID FRIENDLY

DIRECTIONS

Add 5 fresh mint leaves to the bottom of a glass jar, pressing the leaves against the sides of the glass with the back of a spoon to muddle them, releasing their aromatics into the glass.

Place all other ingredients except ice and garnish in the jar and stir well.

Serve over ice with a sprig of fresh mint and a lemon wedge, if desired. Enjoy!

Consume immediately or within 24 hours after straining, if refrigerated.

Drink up to four servings per day.

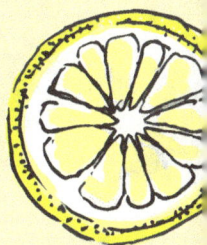

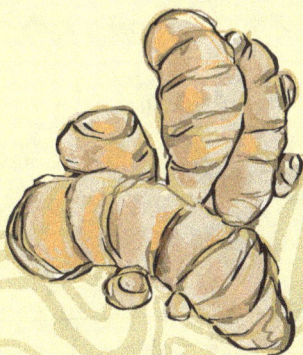

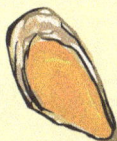

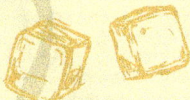

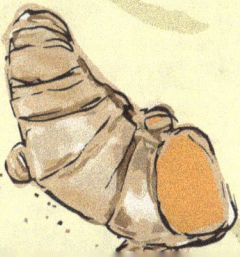

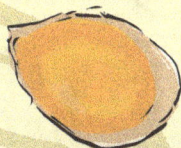

Autumn

Botanical blends that celebrate the flavors of fall produce and warming spices, boost the immune system, and dig into the power of roots.

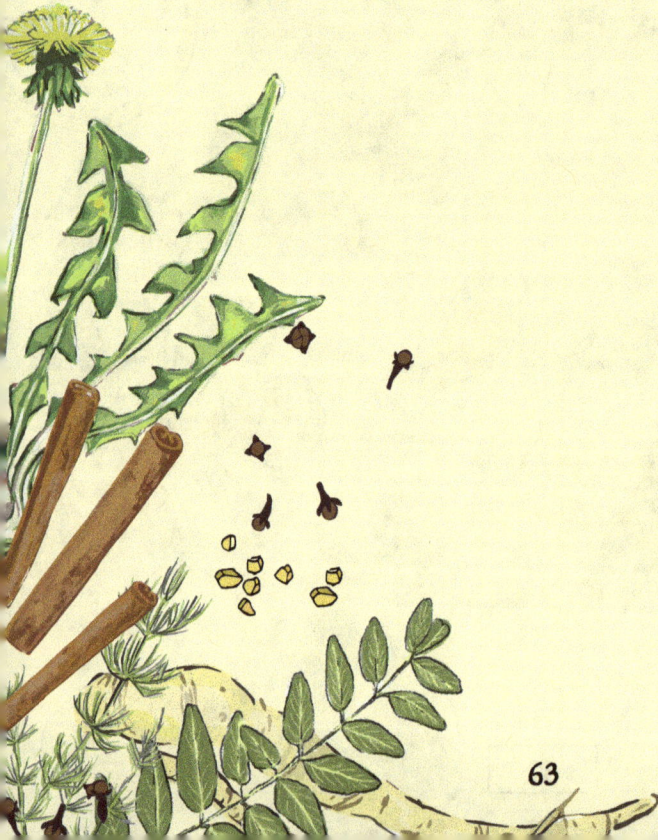

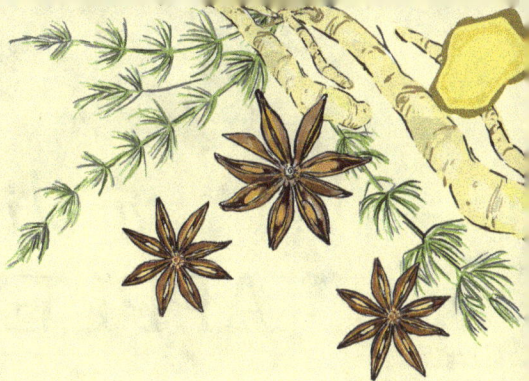

RECIPES:

a slice of
APPLE PIE *tea*

Apple pie tea is a sweet, warm, and exquisite little treat. This tasty tea is a great way to use leftover pie apples or any type of apples before they turn.

Yield: Approximately two 8 fl oz servings

INGREDIENTS

3 fresh apples, sliced

16 fl oz (480 mL) water

2 tbsp (30 mL) honey (or sweetener of choice)

1 tsp cinnamon (*Cinnamomum* spp.) bark, powdered

1 pinch ginger (*Zingiber officinale*) rhizome, powdered

1 pinch clove (*Syzygium aromaticum*) bud, powdered

1 pinch nutmeg (*Myristica fragrans*) seed, powdered, for garnish (optional)

DIRECTIONS

Place sliced apples in a saucepan with water.

Bring to a boil, cover, then reduce the heat to a simmer until the apples are soft.

Remove from heat, strain mixture into a heat-safe container using a tea strainer, and compost or discard fruit material.

Add remaining ingredients and stir well.

Serve with a sprinkle of nutmeg, if desired, and enjoy!.

Consume immediately or within 48 hours after straining, if refrigerated.

Drink up to four servings per day.

| KID FRIENDLY

autumn
ROOT TONIC TRIO

This herbal trio is nourishing and immune supportive, just what the body is seeking as we move into the colder months. As a root-based blend, this combination is a perfect reflection of autumn's harvest of herbal roots, connecting us with seasonal rhythms that nourish us as well. You can make this as a decoction or use the directions below for a long-steeped infusion for a simple, hands-off approach.

Yield: Four 8 fl oz servings

INGREDIENTS

2 tbsp shatavari (*Asparagus racemosus*) root

1 tbsp dandelion (*Taraxacum officinale*) root

1 tbsp astragalus (*Astragalus mongholicus*) root

32 fl oz (960 mL) water

Milk of choice (dairy or non-dairy) (optional)

Honey (or sweetener of choice) to taste (optional)

DIRECTIONS

Place herbs in a heat-safe container.

Pour freshly boiled hot water over the herbs, cover, and steep for 8 hours to overnight.

Strain the infusion through a tea strainer and compost or discard plant material.

Add honey and/or milk, if desired.

Rewarm if desired, serve, and enjoy!

Consume immediately or within 24 hours after straining, if refrigerated.

Drink up to four servings per day.

AUTUMN
transitions tea

This seasonal tea blend with warming, stimulating spices is great for the fall season, particularly as it transitions into winter. The blend also includes chicory root to pull in some cooling energetics for a balanced formula as well as for its liver-stimulating qualities.
- Meagan Visser

Yield: 1¼ cups dried tea blend

INGREDIENTS

¼ cup + 2 tbsp cinnamon (*Cinnamomum* spp.) bark, crushed

¼ cup ginger (*Zingiber officinale*) rhizome

2 tbsp cardamom (*Elettaria cardamomum*) seed

2 tbsp chicory (*Cichorium intybus*) root

2 tbsp pink pepper (*Schinus* spp.) fruit

2 tbsp star anise (*Illicium verum*) seed pod

2 tbsp clove (*Syzygium aromaticum*) bud

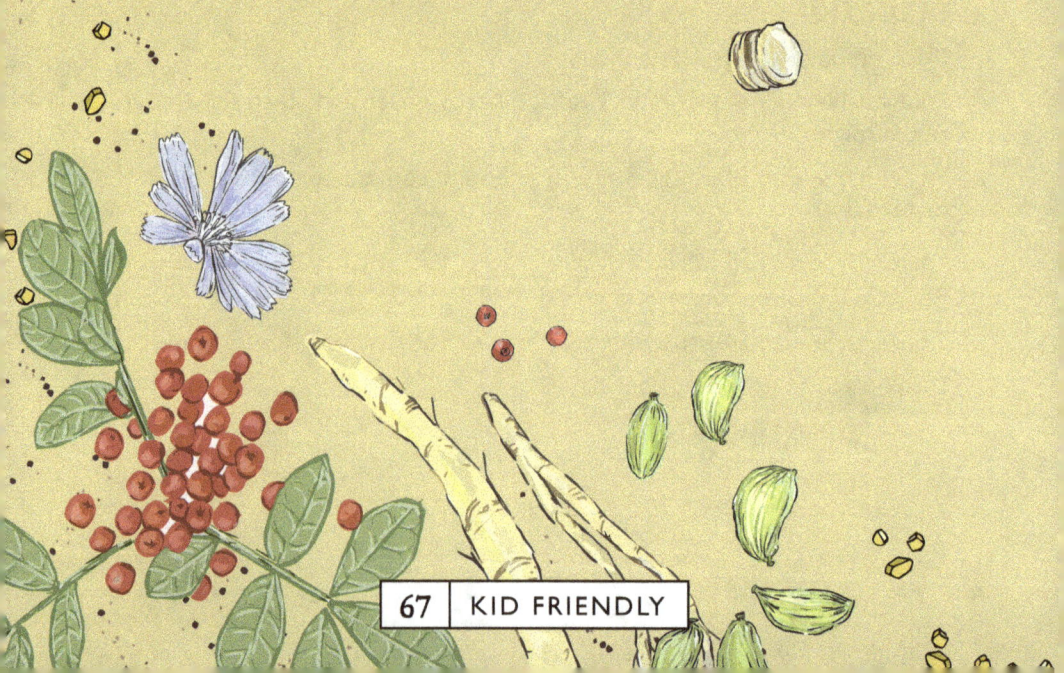

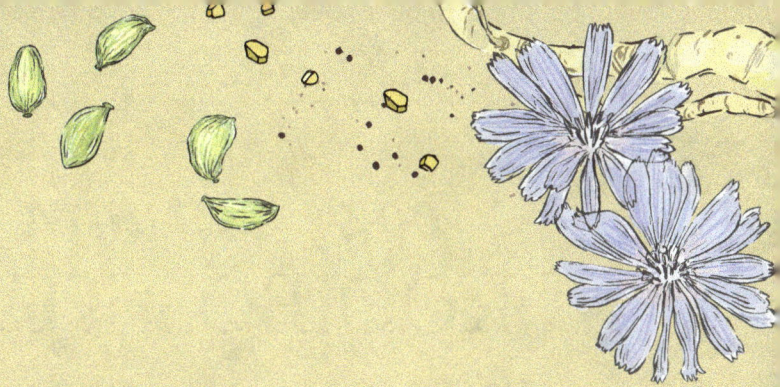

DIRECTIONS

Combine all ingredients and store the blend in a labeled, tightly sealed storage container. Use within 12 months.

Steep 1 tbsp of tea blend per 8 fl oz (240 mL) freshly boiled hot water in a heat-safe container, covered, for 10-15 minutes.

Strain infusion through a tea strainer and compost or discard plant material.

Serve and enjoy!

Drink up to four 8 fl oz servings per day.

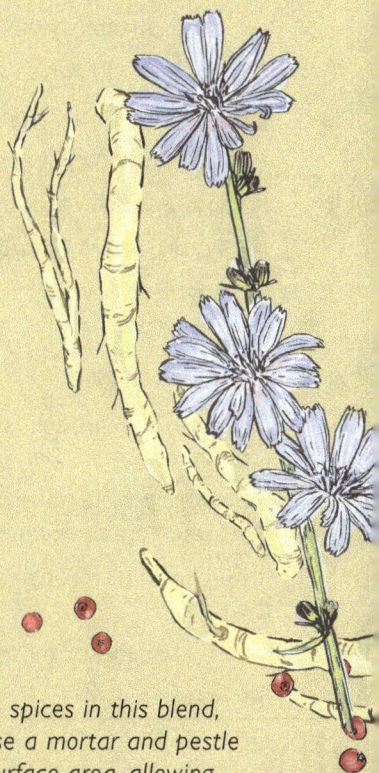

NOTES

If you'd like to enhance the flavor of any of the whole spices in this blend, simply crush them to break them up more. You can use a mortar and pestle or a coffee grinder to do this. This will expose more surface area, allowing more of their volatile oils (hello, flavor and aroma) to be released. However, please don't do this when making your blend, or your spices will lose their flavor more quickly over time! Only do this step when you're getting ready to brew your tea.

cozy autumn
ROOIBOS TEA

With its naturally sweet and nutty flavor, rooibos pairs well with a variety of autumnal spices and tastes. Rich in antioxidants and known to promote heart health, this tea blend not only encapsulates the essence of autumn but also enhances overall wellbeing.

Yield: 1⅛ cup dried tea blend

INGREDIENTS

1 cup red rooibos (*Aspalathus linearis*) leaf

1 tbsp apple (*Malus* spp.) slices, chopped fine

1 tsp orange (*Citrus* spp.) peel, chopped fine

1 stick cinnamon (*Cinnamomum* spp.) bark, crushed

½ tsp clove (*Syzygium aromaticum*) bud, powdered

¼ tsp cardamom (*Elettaria cardamomum*) pod, powdered

¼ tsp ginger (*Zingiber officinale*) rhizome, powdered

DIRECTIONS

Combine all ingredients and store the blend in a labeled, tightly sealed storage container. Use within 12 months.

Steep 1 tsp of tea blend per 8 fl oz (240 mL) freshly boiled hot water in a heat-safe container, covered, for 5-7 minutes.

Strain infusion through a tea strainer and compost or discard plant material.

Add honey and/or milk of choice (dairy or non-dairy), if desired.

Serve and enjoy!

Drink up to four 8 fl oz servings per day.

cup of
PUMPKIN SPICE

Autumn brings about the smell of freshly fallen leaves and pumpkin spice everything! If you are a fan of pumpkin spice, then this tea, incorporating all of the aromatics of the blend, is for you. Add some cream of your choosing and honey to sweeten this cup up. For kids, opt for the caffeine-free tulsi version.

Yield: One 8 fl oz serving

INGREDIENTS

1 tbsp loose black tea (*Camellia sinensis*) leaf (or two tea bags) (or tulsi (*Ocimum tenuiflorum*) aerial parts for a caffeine-free option)

½ tsp ginger (*Zingiber officinale*) rhizome, powdered

¼ tsp cinnamon (*Cinnamomum* spp.) bark, powdered

¼ tsp nutmeg (*Myristica fragrans*) seed, powdered

1 pinch clove (*Syzygium aromaticum*) bud, powdered

8 fl oz (240 mL) water

Milk of choice (dairy or non-dairy) (optional)

Honey (or sweetener of choice) to taste (optional)

DIRECTIONS

Bring water to a simmer in a saucepan, add black tea, cover, and steep for 2 minutes.

Remove from heat, add powdered herbs, and steep for another 2 minutes.

Strain infusion into a heat-safe container using a tea strainer, and compost or discard plant material.

Add honey and/or milk of choice (dairy or non-dairy), if desired.

Drink up to four servings per day.

Pine
+
Cinnamon Tea

Pine and cinnamon create a simple yet potent botanical blend sure to stoke the digestive fire and create warmth on a cold day. Pairing with a bit of honey will add a harmonizing sweetness to this deeply aromatic tea blend.

Yield: Two 8 fl oz servings

INGREDIENTS

3 tbsp fresh pine (*Pinus* spp.) needle, chopped

½ stick cinnamon (*Cinnamomum* spp.) bark, crushed

16 fl oz (480 mL) water

Honey (or sweetener of choice) to taste (optional)

DIRECTIONS

Place herbs in a heat-safe mug or container.

Pour freshly boiled hot water over the herbs, cover, and steep for 20 minutes.

Strain the infusion through a tea strainer and compost or discard plant material.

Sweeten with honey, if desired.

Serve and enjoy!

Consume immediately or within 24 hours after straining, if refrigerated.

Drink up to four servings per day.

ROASTED
root blend

While a hot cup of coffee is the go-to beverage of choice for many, these roasted roots make a wonderfully nourishing morning blend to start the day off right. Chicory and dandelion walk the bitter line with their hint of rooted sweetness, while carob adds a chocolatey layer to the blend.

Yield: 2 cups dried tea blend

INGREDIENTS

1 cup chicory (*Cichorium intybus*) root, roasted

½ cup dandelion (*Taraxacum officinal*) root, roasted

½ cup carob (*Ceratonia siliqua*) pod, roasted

DIRECTIONS

Combine all ingredients and store the blend in a labeled, tightly sealed storage container. Use within 12 months.

Place 1 tbsp of tea blend in a saucepan with 8 fl oz (480 mL) water.

Bring to a boil, cover, then reduce the heat to a simmer.

Simmer for 10-15 minutes, stirringly occasionally.

Remove from heat, and strain infusion into two heat-safe mugs and compost or discard herbal material.

Add milk and sweetener or choice, if desired, and stir well to combine.

Drink up to four 8 fl oz servings per day.

spiced CRANBERRY TEA

Cranberry and cinnamon are quite the autumnal pairing, with an infusion of orange to finish it off with a citrus twist. This blend not only tastes great but is high in antioxidants and is helpful for balancing blood sugar after the indulgence of the season's gatherings.

Yield: Approximately two 8 fl oz servings

INGREDIENTS

1 cup fresh cranberry fruit

1 stick cinnamon (*Cinnamomum* spp.) bark, crushed

1 pinch allspice (*Pimenta dioica*) fruit, powdered

24 fl oz (720 mL) water

Fresh orange, sliced in rounds, for garnish (optional)

DIRECTIONS

Place all ingredients except orange slices in a saucepan.

Bring to a boil, cover, then reduce the heat to a simmer.

Simmer for 20 minutes. Occasionally, use a potato masher or fork to crush the cranberries to release their juice.

Strain decoction into a heat-safe container using a tea strainer, and compost or discard plant material.

Pour into two mugs and place an orange round in each to float on top for garnish.

Drink up to four servings per day.

TULSI
sunrise tea

Tulsi and turmeric pair like a dream and are combined with other aromatic herbs in this sunrise tea blend for a tasty way to start the day (with an added anti-inflammatory boost from turmeric and ginger!). Brew up a cup of this delightful morning tea and go watch the sun rise!

Yield: One 8 fl oz serving

INGREDIENTS

1 tsp tulsi (*Ocimum tenuiflorum*) aerial parts

1 tsp lemongrass (*Cymbopogon citratus*) leaf

½ tsp orange (*Citrus* spp.) peel

¼ tsp turmeric (*Curcuma longa*) rhizome, powdered

¼ tsp ginger (*Zingiber officinalis*) rhizome

8 fl oz (240 mL) water

½ tsp (2.5 mL) lemon juice, freshly squeezed

Honey (or sweetener of choice) to taste (optional)

DIRECTIONS

Place herbs in a heat-safe mug or container.

Pour freshly boiled hot water over the herbs, cover, and steep for 10 minutes.

Strain the infusion through a tea strainer and compost or discard plant material.

Add lemon juice, and sweeten with honey, if desired.

Sip and enjoy!

Drink one serving in the morning.

Winter

Botanical blends that keep us warm and
cozy, provide deep nourishment and
ongoing immune support, and cradle our
hearts and minds with gentleness and calm
that encourage the restorative rest that
winter provides.

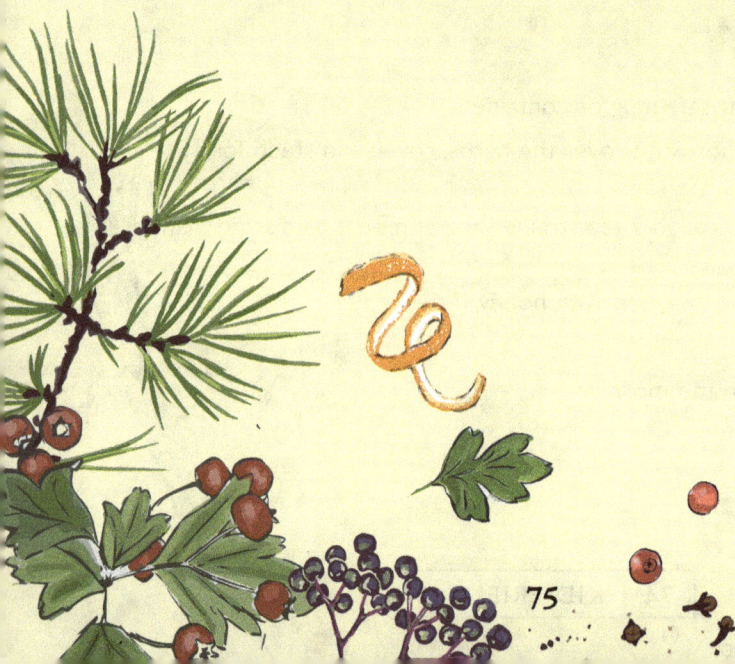

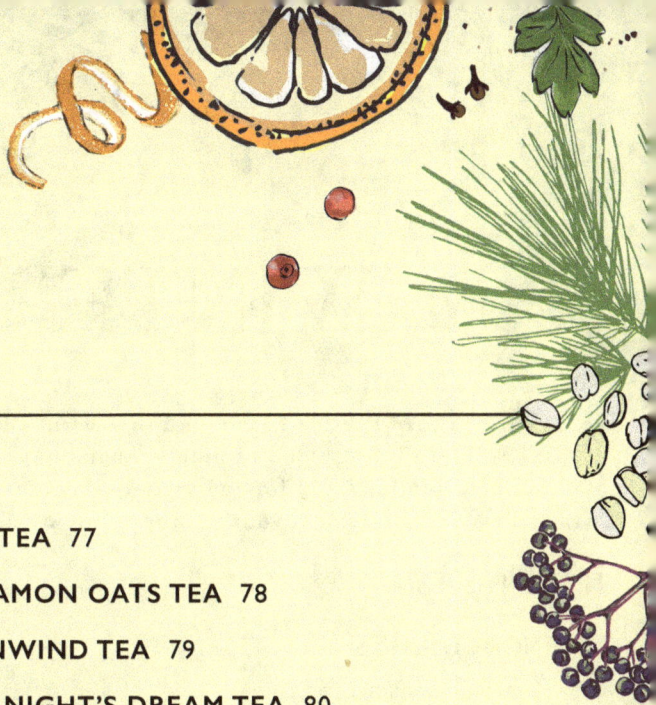

a WINTER'S *tea*

Picture a cozy fireside hearth and this warm cup of gently spiced tea at your side. A blend of pine, cinnamon, and friends is a perfect combination for a comforting winter's day tea. With the nourishing addition of astragalus, your immune system will thank you.

Yield: 1½ cups dried tea blend

INGREDIENTS

¾ cup pine (*Pinus* spp.) needle

¼ cup cinnamon (*Cinnamomum* spp.) bark, crushed

¼ cup astragalus (*Astragalus mongholicus*) root

2 tbsp orange (*Citrus* spp.) peel

2 tbsp clove (*Syzygium aromaticum*) bud

DIRECTIONS

Combine all ingredients and store the blend in a labeled, tightly sealed storage container. Use within 12 months.

Place ¼ cup dried herbal blend in a saucepan with 32 fl oz (960 mL) water.

Bring to a boil, cover, then reduce the heat to a simmer.

Simmer for 20 minutes.

Remove from heat, strain decoction into a heat-safe container using a tea strainer, and compost or discard plant material.

Consume immediately or within 48 hours after straining, if refrigerated.

Drink up to two 8 fl oz servings per day.

cozy
CINNAMON OATS TEA

Reminiscent of a hot breakfast, this tea has the flavor profile of a bowl of oatmeal without the dose of morning starch! The mineral-dense oat straw in this blend provides added nutritive benefits, and along with the blood sugar regulating actions of cinnamon and licorice, this is a truly balanced way to start the day.

Yield: One 8 fl oz serving

INGREDIENTS

1 tbsp oat (*Avena sativa*) straw

¼ tsp cinnamon (*Cinnamomum* spp.) bark, crushed

⅛ tsp licorice (*Glycyrrhiza glabra*) root, powder

8 fl oz (240 mL) water

DIRECTIONS

Place herbs in a heat-safe mug or container.

Pour freshly boiled hot water over the herbs, cover, and steep for 10 minutes.

Strain the infusion through a tea strainer and compost or discard plant material.

Sip and enjoy!

Drink up to two servings per day.

HOLIDAY
unwind tea

The herbs in this calming blend help the body and mind unwind into delightful ease. With its cardioprotective, diuretic, hypotensive, antispasmodic, and nervine actions, this tea also offers balancing support for those with hypertension.

Yield: One 12 fl oz serving

INGREDIENTS

1 tbsp linden (*Tilia* spp.) flower and bract

1 tbsp nettle (*Urtica dioica*) leaf

2 tsp tulsi (*Ocimum tenuiflorum*) aerial parts

1 tsp hawthorn (*Crataegus* spp.) berry, flower, and/or leaf

12 fl oz (360 mL) water

DIRECTIONS

Place herbs in a heat-safe mug or container.

Pour freshly boiled hot water over the herbs, cover, and steep for 10-15 minutes.

Strain the infusion through a tea strainer and compost or discard plant material.

Serve and enjoy!

Drink up to four servings per day.

midwinter night's DREAM TEA

Winter is a time of slowing as the days grow shorter and the nights longer. It invites sleep and dreams, and offers a period where we can welcome in guidance from a long night's rest. This tea blend is filled with herbs that induce dreaming, and when taken before sleep it can help to facilitate lucid dreaming.

Yield: 2 cups dried tea blend

INGREDIENTS

¾ cup ashwagandha (*Withania somnifera*) root, powdered

¾ cup passionflower (*Passiflora incarnata*) aerial parts

¼ cup mugwort (*Artemisia vulgaris*) leaf

¼ cup rosemary (*Salvia rosmarinus*) leaf

DIRECTIONS

Combine all ingredients and store the blend in a labeled, tightly sealed storage container. Use within 12 months.

Steep 2-3 tbsp of tea blend per 8 fl oz (240 mL) freshly boiled hot water in a heat-safe container, covered, for 10-15 minutes.

Strain infusion through a tea strainer and compost or discard plant material.

Drink one 8 fl oz serving 30-60 minutes before bed.

ORANGE
spice tea

Warm up this winter with a circulatory- and immune-stimulating orange spice tea blend. Perfect to sip slowly on a cold winter's day—it will not only bring warmth to your body but it smells and tastes great, too. Not only that, but it's caffeine-free so you can enjoy it day or night without it keeping you awake once you're ready for bed.

Yields: 1⅞ cups dried tea blend

INGREDIENTS

1 cup red rooibos (*Aspalathus linearis*) leaf

½ cup cinnamon (*Cinnamomum* spp.) bark, crushed

¼ cup orange (*Citrus* spp.) peel

2 tbsp clove (*Syzygium aromaticum*) bud

DIRECTIONS

Combine all ingredients and store the blend in a labeled, tightly sealed storage container. Use within 12 months.

Steep 2 tsp of tea blend per 8 fl oz (240 mL) freshly boiled hot water in a heat-safe container, covered, for 10-15 minutes.

Strain infusion through a tea strainer and compost or discard plant material.

Serve and enjoy!

Drink up to four 8 fl oz servings per day.

Waning Moon
herbal tea for
DEEP NOURISHMENT

This easy herbal recipe is made with dried, powdered herbs and is enjoyable in hot water or hot milk of choice. Enjoy this tonifying mix during the waning moon or any time your body, mind, and/or immune system needs a little bolstering.

Yield: 9 tbsp tea blend powder

INGREDIENTS

¼ cup ashwagandha (*Withania somnifera*) root, powdered

2 tbsp astragalus (*Astragalus mongholicus*) root, powdered

2 tbsp hawthorn (*Crataegus* spp.) berry, powdered

1 tbsp ginger (*Zingiber officinale*) rhizome, powdered

DIRECTIONS

Combine all ingredients and store the blend in a labeled, tightly sealed storage container. Use within 12 months.

Place 1 tsp powdered herb blend in a heat-safe mug.

Bring 8 fl oz (240 mL) water to a boil and let cool briefly, then pour over the powdered herbs until the mug is about ¼ full.

Use a whisk or fork to stir briskly for 30 seconds.

Add the remainder of the hot water. If you prefer a latte-style tea, substitute warmed milk of choice (dairy or non-dairy) and stir well to combine.

Sip and enjoy!

Drink up to four 8 fl oz servings per day.

winter solstice HEART TEA

Formulated to lighten the heart with herbs that encourage openings, this tea was designed to be sipped under the moon on the winter solistic's night. Welcome the lengthening of the days with this tea blend for a solstice evening ritual.

Yield: Approximately one 8 fl oz serving

INGREDIENTS

1 tbsp hawthorn (*Crataegus* spp.) berry

2 tsp rose (*Rosa* spp.) petal

¼ tsp cinnamon (*Cinnamomum* spp.) bark, crushed

16 fl oz (480 mL) water

DIRECTIONS

Place hawthorn in a saucepan with water.

Bring to a boil, cover, then reduce the heat to a simmer.

Simmer for 20 minutes.

Remove from heat, add rose and cinnamon, cover, and steep for 10 minutes.

Strain decoction into a heat-safe container using a tea strainer, and compost or discard plant material.

Drink up to two servings per day.

WINTER SPICE TEA

This warming tea is not only tasty, but it also contains herbs rich in vitamin C and other immune-boosting compounds that can help keep wintertime respiratory infections at bay.

Yield: Four 8 fl oz servings

INGREDIENTS

2 tbsp cinnamon (*Cinnamomum* spp.) bark, crushed

1 tbsp rose (*Rosa* spp.) hip

2 tsp orange (*Citrus* spp.) peel

2 tsp elder (*Sambucus nigra* or *S. canadensis*) berry

1 tsp ginger (*Zingiber officinale*) rhizome

32 fl oz (960 mL) water

DIRECTIONS

Place herbs in a heat-safe container.

Pour freshly boiled hot water over the herbs, cover, and steep for 25-30 minutes.

Strain the infusion through a tea strainer and compost or discard plant material.

Serve and enjoy!

Consume immediately or within 24 hours after straining, if refrigerated.

Drink up to four servings per day.

winter
TONIC TEA

A warming, flavorful tea with tonic herbs and spicy notes to enliven digestion and circulation. Adaptogenic tulsi will melt the stressors of the winter season away, while hawthorn nourishes the heart. Cinnamon and ginger add flavor, warmth, and the aromatic benefits of these herbs. Try this tonic blend on any winter's day. If including licorice, short term use is suggested.

Yield: One 12 fl oz serving

INGREDIENTS

2 tsp tulsi (*Ocimum tenuiflorum*) aerial parts

½ tsp cinnamon (*Cinnamomum* spp.) bark, crushed

½ tsp ginger (*Zingiber officinale*) rhizome

1 tsp hawthorn (*Crataegus* spp.) berry (optional)

¼ tsp licorice (*Glycyrrhiza glabra*) root (optional)

12 fl oz (360 mL) water

DIRECTIONS

Place herbs in a heat-safe container.

Pour freshly boiled hot water over the herbs, cover, and steep for 10-15 minutes.

Strain the infusion through a tea strainer and compost or discard plant material.

Serve and enjoy!

Drink up to two servings per day.

Tea is a wonderful support for the mind and spirit... Take for instance the way the warm cup feels in your hands, or the sight of the steam curling upwards to caress your skin when taking those first sips.

HERBAL ACADEMY'S
TEA BLENDING 101 MINI COURSE

CHAPTER FOUR
WELLNESS TEAS

It will come as no surprise that botanical tea blends are a staple preparation for utilizing herbs to support our wellness! A cup of tea is an easy and accessible way to incorporate herbs into our daily routines, with the added benefit of being a beautifully grounding practice for the mind and spirit. The process of creating a tea blend and preparing the tea, as well as holding the cup in our hands, inhaling the steam, tasting the interplay of flavors on our tongue, and tuning in to the tea's actions throughout our body is a delightfully nourishing benefit of consuming herbs in this manner.

In this chapter, you will find wellness-focused herbal tea blends for a wide variety of needs for which many of us seek support. We've grouped these into the following categories:

Calm and Ground – Botanical blends that soothe and ground the nervous system, invite delight and uplift the spirit, lull us into a dreamy sleep, care for a broken heart, and provide the nurturing support we all deserve.

Digest and Cleanse – Botanical blends that support and optimize the digestive process, calm post-meal upset, soothe gut tissues, nourish and tone the organs of elimination, and support skin health.

Energize and Uplift - Botanical blends that boost energy, sharpen mental focus and clarity, put a delightful pep in our step, invite creativity and enchantment, offer solace, and support self love.

Generate and Eliminate - Botanical blends that address common complaints in the urinary and reproductive systems, easing uncomfortable symptoms, and ensuring smooth function.

Nourish and Strengthen - Botanical blends that offer adaptogens to support the body's stress response, antioxidants to optimize the cardiovascular system, minerals to strengthen the bones, and nourishing nutrients for tip-top function throughout the body.

Protect and Soothe - Botanical blends that support healthy immune function, provide a boost when you're starting to feel under the weather, ease a sore throat, get congestion moving, calm a cough, and soothe a fever.

SECTIONS:

Calm & Ground

Botanical blends that soothe and ground
the nervous system, invite delight and
uplift the spirit, lull us into a dreamy
sleep, care for a broken heart, and provide
the nurturing support we all deserve.

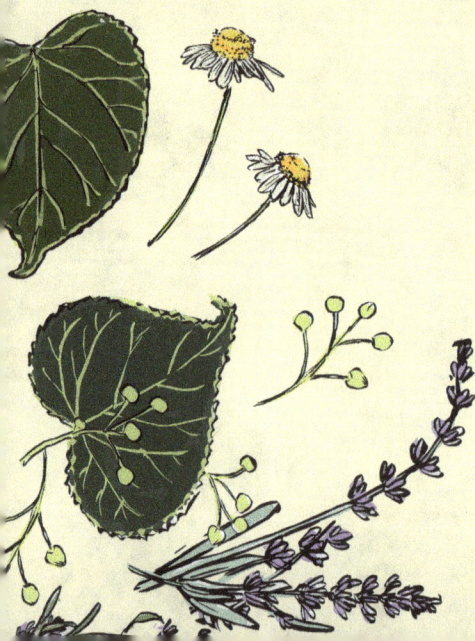

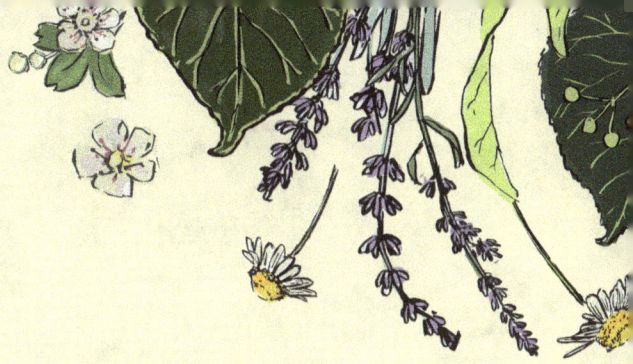

RECIPES:

AVIVA ROMM'S
Gentle Evening Tea

Dr. Aviva Romm—physician, herbalist, mother, and midwife—shared this calming tea blend with our Herbal Academy community. And what a treat! In this simple blend, Aviva includes three familiar herbs for a gentle and lovely tea that makes every evening a celebration.

Yield: One 8 fl oz serving

INGREDIENTS

1 tsp chamomile (*Matricaria chamomilla*) flower

1 tsp lavender (*Lavandula* spp.) flower bud

1 tsp peppermint (*Mentha x piperita*) leaf

8 fl oz (240 mL) water

DIRECTIONS

Place herbs in a heat-safe mug or container.

Pour freshly boiled hot water over the herbs, cover, and steep for 3-5 minutes.

Strain the infusion through a tea strainer and compost or discard plant material.

Sip and enjoy!

Drink one serving in the evening.

Blissful Being Tea

This herbal tea blend is full of nerve-soothing plant allies. Perfect for the evening, late afternoon, or any time your nervous system needs a little smoothing out, the overall cool energy of this tea makes it especially suitable for *pitta dosha*. Gotu kola is a *pitta*-pacifying nervine that supports a calm, cool, and collected mind. This blend may also be quite helpful for *vata* types who tend toward nervousness and sleep troubles.

Yield: 1¼ cups dried tea blend

INGREDIENTS

½ cup gotu kola (*Centella asiatica*) leaf

½ cup tulsi (*Ocimum tenuiflorum*) aerial parts

1 tbsp lavender (*Lavandula* spp.) flower bud

1 tbsp skullcap (*Scutellaria lateriflora*) aerial parts

1 tbsp lemon balm (*Melissa officinalis*) aerial parts

1 tbsp chamomile (*Matricaria chamomilla*) flower

DIRECTIONS

Combine all ingredients and store the blend in a labeled, tightly sealed storage container. Use within 12 months.

Steep 1 tbsp of tea blend per 8 fl oz (240 mL) freshly boiled hot water in a heat-safe container, covered, for 20 minutes.

Strain infusion through a tea strainer and compost or discard plant material.

Sip and enjoy!

Drink up to four servings per day.

CALM
+ STEADY TEA

Keep calm and support your nervous system when it feels a bit on edge or frazzled with this botanical tea intended to soothe and support you when you need it most.

Yield: One 12 fl oz serving

INGREDIENTS

2 tsp skullcap (*Scutellaria lateriflora*) aerial parts

1½ tsp damiana (*Turnera diffusa*) aerial parts

1 tsp linden (*Tilia* spp.) bract and flower

1 tsp lavender (*Lavandula* spp.) flower bud

12 fl oz (360 mL) water

Milk of choice (dairy or non-dairy) (optional)

Honey (or sweetener of choice) (optional)

DIRECTIONS

Place herbs in a heat-safe container.

Pour freshly boiled hot water over the herbs, cover, and steep for 10-15 minutes.

Strain the infusion through a tea strainer and compost or discard plant material.

Add milk of choice (dairy or non-dairy) and sweeten with honey (or sweetener of choice) to taste, if desired.

Serve and enjoy!

Drink up to four servings per day.

Calming LINDEN TEA

Enjoy a mug of this tasty herbal tea 30-60 minutes before bed or anytime a little calm is needed. Loaded with relaxing nervine herbs, this botanical beverage will help settle your spirits in no time.

Yield: One 8 fl oz serving

INGREDIENTS

2 tsp linden (*Tilia* spp.) flower and bract

I tsp spearmint (*Mentha spicata*) leaf

I tsp calendula (*Calendula officinalis*) flower

½ tsp catnip (*Nepeta cataria*) aerial parts

½ tsp lavender (*Lavandula* spp.) flower bud

8 fl oz (240 mL) water

DIRECTIONS

Place herbs in a heat-safe container.

Pour freshly boiled hot water over the herbs, cover, and steep for 15-30 minutes.

Strain the infusion through a tea strainer and compost or discard plant material.

Serve and enjoy!

Drink up to four servings per day.

Calming TEA

This blend of nervine herbs comes from our Herbal Stress Management course, which delves into the holistic approach to self care for stress management and provides insight into helpful nutritional choices, lifestyle practices, and herbs that can transform your response to stress and enhance your wellbeing.

Yield: 1⅜ cups dried tea blend

INGREDIENTS

½ cup lemon balm (*Melissa officinalis*) aerial parts

¼ cup chamomile (*Matricaria chamomilla*) flower

¼ cup linden (*Tilia* spp.) flower and bract

¼ cup rose (*Rosa* spp.) petal

2 tbsp spearmint (*Mentha spicata*) leaf

DIRECTIONS

Combine all ingredients and store the blend in a labeled, tightly sealed storage container. Use within 12 months.

Steep 1-2 tbsp of tea blend per 8 fl oz (240 mL) freshly boiled hot water in a heat-safe container, covered, for 10-15 minutes.

Strain infusion through a tea strainer and compost or discard plant material.

Serve and enjoy!

Drink up to four 8 fl oz servings per day.

CALMING
Quartet Tea

When you feel your muscles begin to tighten and clench up, call upon the stress-soothing properties of this quartet of botanicals to ease tension, relax muscles, and soothe frayed nerves.

Yield: One 8 fl oz serving

INGREDIENTS

1 tsp skullcap (*Scutellaria lateriflora*) aerial parts

1 tsp chamomile (*Matricaria chamomilla*) flower

½ tsp motherwort (*Leonurus cardiaca*) aerial parts

½ tsp rose (*Rosa* spp.) petal

8 fl oz (240 mL) water

1 sprig fresh mint (*Mentha* spp.) or slice fresh ginger (*Zingiber officinale*) rhizome, for garnish (optional)

DIRECTIONS

Place all herbs except garnish in a heat-safe container.

Pour freshly boiled hot water over the herbs, cover, and steep for 5 minutes.

Strain the infusion through a tea strainer and compost or discard plant material.

Serve with a sprig of fresh mint or a slice of fresh ginger, if desired, and enjoy!

Drink up to four servings per day.

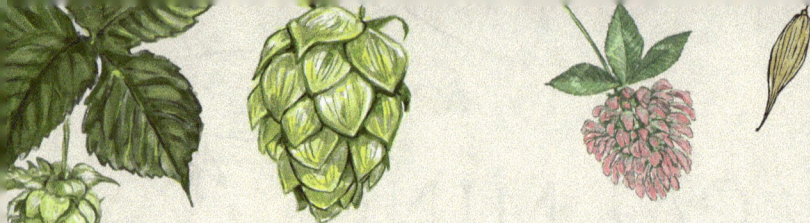

CLOUD NINE TEA

An herbal cloud to carry your troubles away, this nourishing and relaxing blend is designed to cultivate rest and restoration, and is best made when there is little to do but sip tea, take deep breaths, and gaze at the sky.
- Lindsey Feldpausch

Yield: Two 8 fl oz servings

INGREDIENTS

1 tbsp hops (*Humulus lupulus*) strobile

2 tsp oat (*Avena sativa*) milky seed or straw

2 tsp red clover (*Trifolium pratense*) aerial parts

1 tsp lemon balm (*Melissa officinalis*) aerial parts

16 fl oz (480 mL) water

DIRECTIONS

Place herbs in a heat-safe container.

Pour freshly boiled hot water over the herbs, cover, and steep for 15-20 minutes.

Strain the infusion through a tea strainer and compost or discard plant material.

Serve and enjoy!

Drink up to four servings per day.

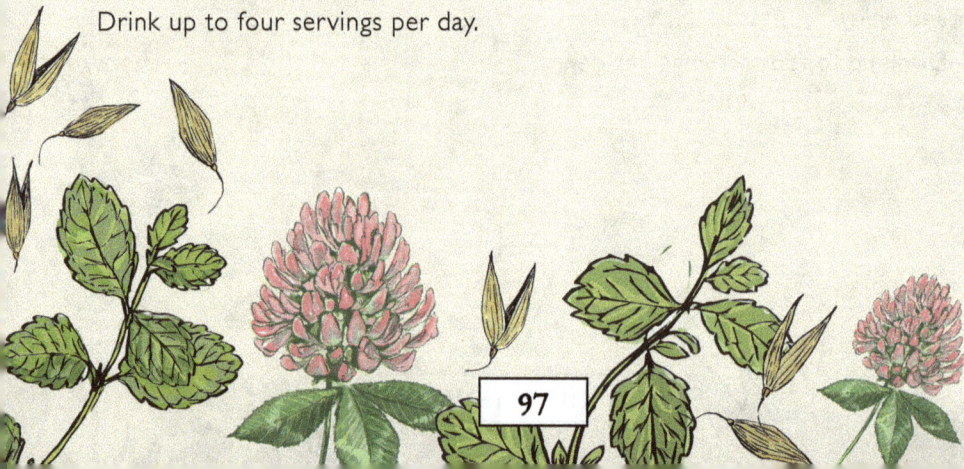

FAIRY
QUEEN TEA

An aromatic floral tea blend that is surely enjoyed by the fairy queen herself. This tea is quick to prepare and light and airy, yet grounding. Let it soothe your afternoon cares away! Best sipped under the shade of a favorite tree. For kids and if desired in pregnancy, opt for the caffeine-free nettle version.
- Christie Clark

Yield: One 8 fl oz serving

INGREDIENTS

1 tsp white or green tea (*Camellia sinensis*) leaf (or nettle (*Urtica dioica*) leaf for a caffeine-free option)

½ tsp chamomile (*Matricaria chamomilla*) flower

½ tsp rose (*Rosa* spp.) petal

8 fl oz (240 mL) water

Honey (or sweetener of choice) to taste (optional)

DIRECTIONS

Place herbs in a heat-safe container.

Pour freshly boiled hot water over the herbs, cover, and steep for 3-5 minutes.

Strain the infusion through a tea strainer and compost or discard plant material.

Sweeten with honey, if desired.

Serve and enjoy!

Drink up to four servings per day.

GROUNDING
Gratitude Tea

Tune in and ground down with this herbal tea blend. Equally spotlighting the adaptogenic tulsi and nourishing bitter dandelion, paired with a bit of ginger to increase movement, this recipe can be used in the grounding practice of your choosing to help you direct energy and flow.

Yield: One 8 fl oz serving

INGREDIENTS

1 tsp tulsi (*Ocimum tenuiflorum*) aerial parts

1 tsp dandelion (*Taraxacum officinale*) root

½ tsp ginger (*Zingiber officinale*) rhizome (or 2 fresh ginger slices, sliced thinly)

8 fl oz (240 mL) water

DIRECTIONS

Place herbs in a heat-safe container.

Pour freshly boiled hot water over the herbs, cover, and steep for 15-20 minutes.

Strain the infusion through a tea strainer and compost or discard plant material.

Serve and enjoy!

Drink up to four servings per day.

Heart's Ease Tea

A blend of plant allies to soothe and support the heart, both energetically and physically. Not only do the plants in this blend nourish and soothe the emotional heart, helping to ease feelings of stress and anxiety, but they are all known for their cardiovascular-supportive properties.

Yield: Two 8 fl oz servings

INGREDIENTS

1 tbsp linden (*Tilia* spp.) flower and bract

2 tsp violet (*Viola odorata* or *V. sororia*) flower

1 tsp skullcap (*Scutellaria lateriflora*) aerial parts

1 tsp hawthorn (*Crataegus* spp.) leaf, flower, and/or berry

1 tsp rose (*Rosa* spp.) petal

1 cardamom (*Elettaria cardamomum*) pod, crushed

16 fl oz (480 mL) water

DIRECTIONS

Place herbs in a heat-safe container.

Pour freshly boiled hot water over the herbs, cover, and steep for 10-15 minutes.

Strain the infusion through a tea strainer and compost or discard plant material.

Serve and enjoy!

Drink up to four servings per day.

Grief Solace tea

Grief comes in many shapes and forms, but no matter how you experience it, bringing along your herbal allies can be supportive. This combination of nurturing nervines is crafted to instill a feeling of heart opening and acceptance that won't stop the emotions but, instead, let them flow through you. Reach for this blend when you need an herbal friend.

Yield: Two 8 fl oz servings

INGREDIENTS

2 tsp violet (*Viola odorata* or *V. sororia*) leaf

1 tsp motherwort (*Leonurus cardiaca*) aerial parts

1 tsp rose (*Rosa* spp.) petal

1 tsp hawthorn (*Crataegus* spp.) berry

1 tsp linden (*Tilia* spp.) flower and bract

½ tsp cinnamon (*Cinnamomum* spp.) bark, crushed

1 cardamom (*Elettaria cardamomum*) pod, crushed

16 fl oz (480 mL) water

DIRECTIONS

Place herbs in a heat-safe container.

Pour freshly boiled hot water over the herbs, cover, and steep for 5-7 minutes.

Strain the infusion through a tea strainer and compost or discard herbal material.

Serve and enjoy!

Drink up to two servings per day.

KID FRIENDLY

KEEP CALM TEA

Some days there's no going back to bed and trying again tomorrow—you just have to trudge through. If you find yourself having one of those days, this nerve-nourishing tea blend is a great companion to help you get through the day. Not only does it help to settle a frazzled spirit, but it can help to uplift it at the same time.

Yield: 1⅞ cups dried tea blend

INGREDIENTS

½ cup lemon balm (*Melissa officinalis*) aerial parts

½ cup oat (*Avena sativa*) milky seed

½ cup peppermint (*Mentha x piperita*) leaf

¼ cup catnip (*Nepeta cataria*) aerial parts

2 tbsp chamomile (*Matricaria chamomilla*) flower

DIRECTIONS

Combine all ingredients and store the blend in a labeled, tightly sealed storage container. Use within 12 months.

Steep 1 tbsp of tea blend per 8 fl oz (240 mL) freshly boiled hot water in a heat-safe container, covered, for 5-7 minutes.

Strain infusion through a tea strainer and compost or discard plant material.

Sip hot, or allow to cool and serve over ice with 2-3 fresh peppermint leaves.

Drink up to four 8 fl oz servings per day.

Linden
love tea

This tea blend, filled with heart opening and uplifting nervines, can aid in bodily relaxation while calming an agitated or anxious mind, allowing a person to unwind. When consumed before bed, it will aid a gentle ease into slumber and support a peaceful night's sleep. If you try this blend, you may just fall in love with linden!

Yield: 1¼ cups dried tea blend

INGREDIENTS

½ cup linden (*Tilia* spp.) flower and bract

¼ cup rose (*Rosa* spp.) petal

¼ cup chamomile (*Matricaria chamomilla*) flower

¼ cup lemon balm (*Melissa officinalis*) aerial parts

1 pinch cardamom (*Elettaria cardamomum*) seed, powdered

DIRECTIONS

Combine all ingredients and store the blend in a labeled, tightly sealed storage container. Use within 12 months.

Steep 1 tbsp of tea blend per 8 fl oz (240 mL) freshly boiled hot water in a heat-safe container, covered, for 5 minutes.

Strain infusion through a tea strainer and compost or discard plant material.

Serve and enjoy!

Drink up to four 8 fl oz servings per day.

Meadowsweet Tea
with rose

Meadowsweet is a go-to choice for stress-related headaches. Rose (*Rosa* spp.) petals are aromatic, calming, and a gentle nervine perfect for times when you need a little nurturing. For extra flavor, a dash of cardamom and a little sweetener make this a truly pleasant cup of tea.

Yield: One 8 fl oz serving

INGREDIENTS

1 tsp meadowsweet (*Filipendula ulmaria*) flower

1 tsp rose (*Rosa* spp.) petal

1 pinch cardamom (*Elettaria cardamomum*) seed, powdered

8 fl oz (240 mL) water

Honey (or sweetener of choice) to taste (optional)

DIRECTIONS

Place herbs in a heat-safe container.

Pour freshly boiled hot water over the herbs, cover, and steep for 10 minutes.

Strain the infusion through a tea strainer and compost or discard plant material.

Sweeten with honey, if desired.

Serve and enjoy!

Drink up to four servings per day.

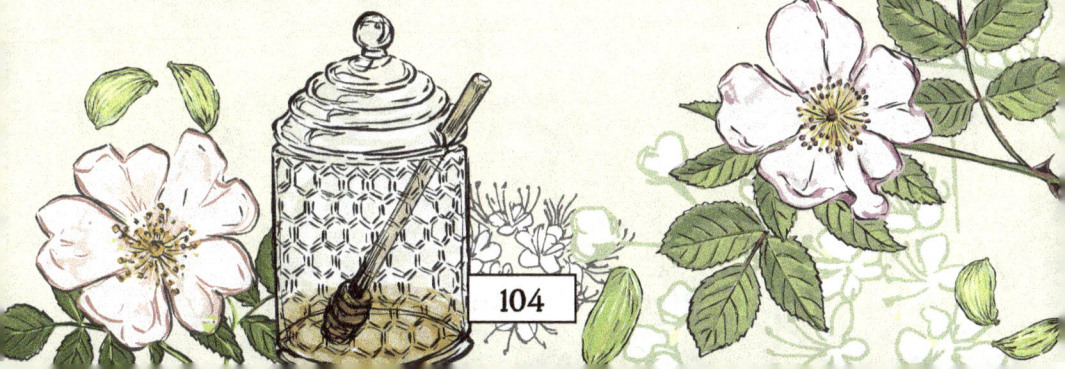

Nerve
BUILDING TEA

Commuter traffic, late nights, screen time, and constant adulting tasks can make your nervous system feel a bit "frayed" over time. Integrating a daily herbal tea can help nourish and restore an overstimulated nervous system.

Yield: 1⅜ cups dried tea blend

INGREDIENTS

½ cup oat (*Avena sativa*) straw

¼ cup violet (*Viola odorata* or *V. sororia*) leaf and/or flower

¼ cup tulsi (*Ocimum tenuiflorum*) aerial parts

¼ cup marshmallow (*Althaea officinalis*) root

2 tbsp skullcap (*Scutellaria lateriflora*) aerial parts

DIRECTIONS

Combine all ingredients and store the blend in a labeled, tightly sealed storage container. Use within 12 months.

Steep 1 tbsp of tea blend per 8 fl oz (240 mL) freshly boiled hot water in a heat-safe container, covered, for 15 minutes.

Strain infusion through a tea strainer and compost or discard plant material.

Serve and enjoy!

Drink up to four 8 fl oz servings per day.

ROSE **RED** TEA

Just like the fairy tale, this Rose Red Tea blend speaks to the lover, the wanderer, the friend, and the helper in all of us. Tightening and toning to the tissues and supportive of the nerves, this tea evokes feelings of love, warmth, heartfelt emotion, and goodwill, even on the coldest of days.

Yield: 2 cups dried tea blend

INGREDIENTS

1 cup red rooibos (*Aspalathus linearis*) leaf

½ cup rose (*Rosa* spp.) petal

¼ cup oat (*Avena sativa*) milky seed

¼ cup rose (*Rosa* spp.) hip

DIRECTIONS

Combine all ingredients and store the blend in a labeled, tightly sealed storage container. Use within 12 months.

Steep 1 tbsp of tea blend per 8 fl oz (240 mL) freshly boiled hot water in a heat-safe container, covered, for 5-10 minutes.

Strain infusion through a tea strainer and compost or discard plant material.

Serve and enjoy!

Drink up to three 8 fl oz servings per day.

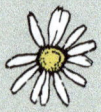

Soothing SLEEP TEA

Whether you have trouble falling asleep, or you spend nights staying awake with anxious thoughts, this blend will help support a good night's rest. Enjoy 30-60 minutes before bedtime and combine with a calming activity such as reading.

Yield: 1¾ cups dried tea blend

INGREDIENTS

1 cup chamomile (*Matricaria chamomilla*) flower

½ cup lemon balm (*Melissa officinalis*) aerial parts

¼ cup rose (*Rosa* spp.) petal

1 tbsp lavender (*Lavandula officinalis*) flower bud

DIRECTIONS

Combine all ingredients and store the blend in a labeled, tightly sealed storage container. Use within 12 months.

Steep 1 tbsp of tea blend per 8 fl oz (240 mL) freshly boiled hot water in a heat-safe container, covered, for 5-7 minutes.

Strain infusion through a tea strainer and compost or discard plant material.

Serve and enjoy!

Drink one 8 fl oz serving 30-60 minutes before bed.

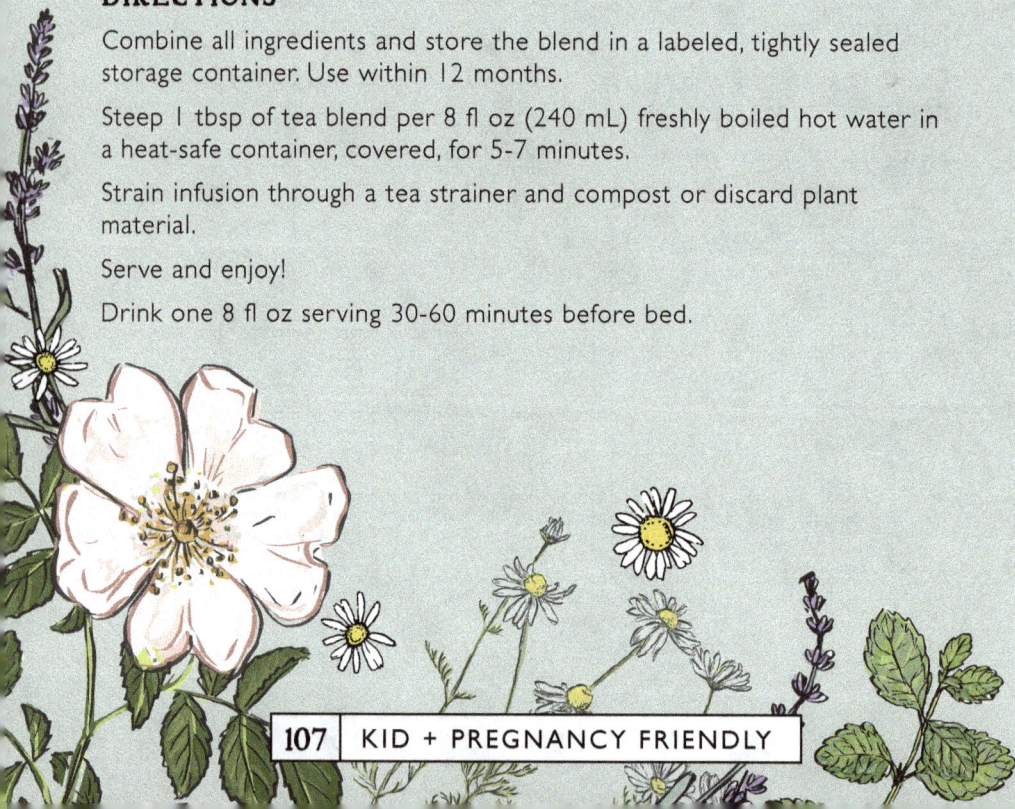

SOOTHING
Nighttime Tea

Relax the body with a cup of this tea an hour before bed so you can drift off to sleep. Filled with relaxing nervines and sedative herbs, this brew will soothe the body and mind so your slumber is a bit sweeter.

Yield: 1⅛ cups dried tea blend

INGREDIENTS

¼ cup chamomile (*Matricaria chamomilla*) flower

¼ cup tulsi (*Ocimum tenuiflorum*) aerial parts

¼ cup lemon balm (*Melissa officinalis*) aerial parts

2 tbsp passionflower (*Passiflora incarnata*) aerial parts

2 tbsp spearmint (*Mentha spicata*) leaf (optional)

2 tbsp orange (*Citrus* spp.) peel

1½ tsp licorice (*Glycyrrhiza glabra*) root (optional)

DIRECTIONS

Combine all ingredients and store the blend in a labeled, tightly sealed storage container. Use within 12 months.

Steep 1 tbsp of tea blend per 8 fl oz (240 mL) freshly boiled hot water in a heat-safe container, covered, for 15-20 minutes.

Strain infusion through a tea strainer and compost or discard plant material.

Serve and enjoy!

Drink one 8 fl oz serving 30-60 minutes before bed.

Digest & Cleanse

Botanical blends that support and optimize the digestive process, calm post-meal upset, soothe gut tissues, nourish and tone the organs of elimination, and support skin health.

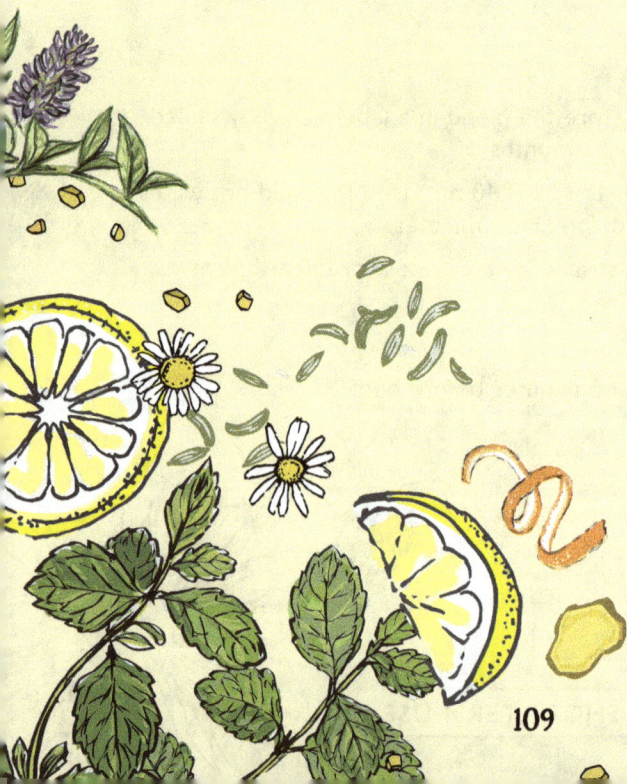

RECIPES:

Abuelita's WILD TEA

My great-grandmother, a well-known *curandera* (traditional healer) in Old Town Albuquerque, would prepare this native herb found throughout the Southwest. She would prepare the tea to be used for the kidneys and stomach aches, and served it as a refreshing drink in the summer. It goes by many names in traditional languages and is also known simply as "wild tea;" however, I grew up knowing it as cota. When I learned to harvest cota in Canyon de Chelly many years ago, the elders taught me to gather it in the way of my ancestors, who would bundle it with flowers and all, to be simmered in a pot of water. It has a delicious, mild flavor and reminds me of my *abuela*. If you cannot source dried bundles, simply substitute 2 teaspoons of broken stems and flowers. In my family, we save the bundle and use it a second time for another round of weaker tea.
- Felicia Cocotzin Ruiz

Yield: Approximately four 8 fl oz servings

INGREDIENTS

1 small bundle cota (*Thelesperma megapotamicum*) aboveground parts (2 tsp garbled aboveground parts)

32 fl oz (960 mL) water

Honey (or sweetener of choice) to taste

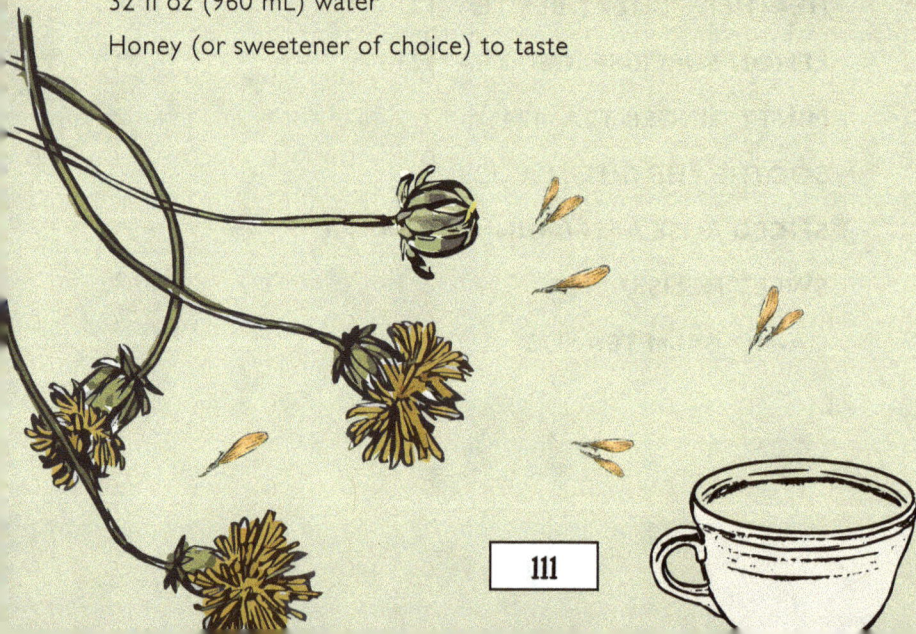

DIRECTIONS

Place cota in a saucepan with water.

Bring to a boil, cover, then reduce the heat to a simmer.

Simmer for 5-10 minutes.

Remove from heat, strain infusion into a heat-safe container using a tea strainer, and compost or discard plant material (or set aside for a second round of weaker tea).

Sweeten with honey, if desired.

Serve hot or allow to cool and enjoy!

Consume immediately or within 24 hours after straining, if refrigerated.

Drink up to four servings per day.

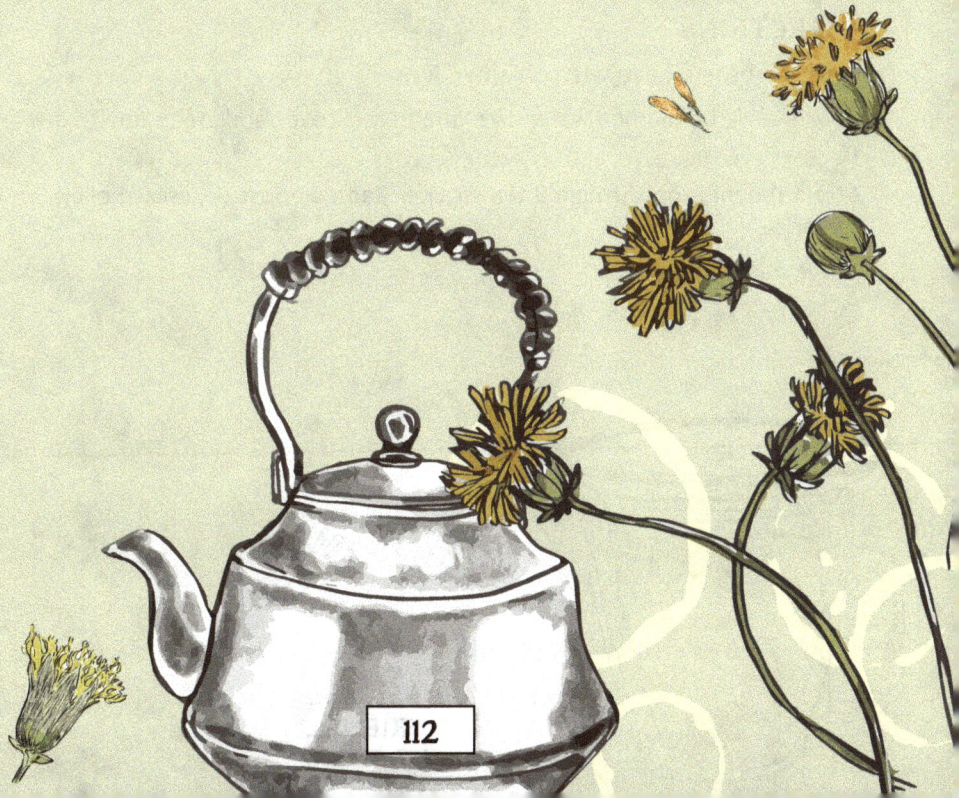

AFTER DINNER
Fennel Tea Recipe

Perhaps the only thing that's better than the gentleness with which fennel helps our digestive processes is the simplicity of how we can enjoy its benefits. The following delicious tea recipe comes from our Intermediate Herbal Course's Digestive System unit.

Yield: One 8 fl oz serving

INGREDIENTS

1 tbsp chamomile (*Matricaria chamomilla*) flower

1 ½ tsp bee balm (*Monarda fistulosa* or *M. didyma*) aerial parts

½ tsp orange (*Citrus* spp.) peel

½ tsp fennel (*Foeniculum vulgare*) seed, powdered

8 fl oz (240 mL) water

DIRECTIONS

Place herbs in a heat-safe container.

Pour freshly boiled hot water over the herbs, cover, and steep for 5-10 minutes.

Strain the infusion through a tea strainer and compost or discard plant material.

Serve and enjoy!

Drink one serving after dinner.

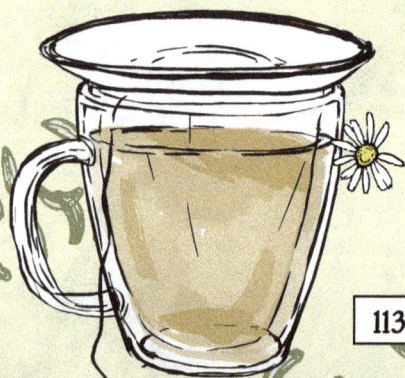

KID FRIENDLY

BITTER TONIC TEA

Embrace the benefits of bitters, from digestive and liver support to tightening and toning of the gut lining, mood support, and more! This tea is meant to be bitter tasting and is best sipped in small quantities twice a day.

Yield: 1½ cups dried tea blend

INGREDIENTS

½ cup roasted dandelion (*Taraxacum officinale*) root

½ cup lemon (*Citrus x limon*) peel

½ cup motherwort (*Leonurus cardiaca*) aerial parts

DIRECTIONS

Combine all ingredients and store the blend in a labeled, tightly sealed storage container. Use within 12 months.

Steep 1 tbsp of tea blend per 8 fl oz (240 mL) freshly boiled hot water in a heat-safe container, covered, for 10 minutes.

Strain infusion through a tea strainer and compost or discard plant material.

Serve and enjoy!

Drink one 4 fl oz serving twice a day.

Clear Skin Tea

Skin issues can lower your confidence level quickly, so if you're struggling with breakouts, discoloration, or patchiness, this botanical tea blend can help support a healthy gut, liver, and lymphatic system—three areas of the body linked to skin health.

Yield: 1¾ cup dried tea blend

INGREDIENTS

½ cup goldenrod (*Solidago* spp.) aerial parts

½ cup calendula (*Calendula officinalis*) flower

½ cup red clover (*Trifolium pratense*) aerial parts

3½ tsp burdock (*Arctium lappa*) root

1½ tsp licorice (*Glycyrrhiza glabra*) root

DIRECTIONS

Combine all ingredients and store the blend in a labeled, tightly sealed storage container. Use within 12 months.

Place ¼ cup tea blend in a saucepan with 40 fl oz (1.2 L) of water.

Bring to a boil, cover, then reduce the heat to a simmer.

Simmer for 20 minutes.

Remove from heat, strain decoction into a heat-safe container using a tea strainer, and compost or discard plant material.

Consume immediately or within 48 hours after straining, if refrigerated.

Drink up to four 8 fl oz servings per day.

CINNAMON APPLE
Mock-Digestif Tea

Settle digestion after a rich meal with this alcohol-free digestif. This tea blend contains carminative herbs that help aid digestion, ease gas and bloating, and soothe spasms in the gastrointestinal tract. It also has a great flavor that will pleasantly surprise your tastebuds.

Yield: 1⅛ cups dried tea blend

INGREDIENTS

½ cup chamomile (*Matricaria chamomilla*) flower

½ cup cinnamon (*Cinnamomum* spp.) bark, crushed

2 tbsp dried apple slices, chopped fine

DIRECTIONS

Combine all ingredients and store the blend in a labeled, tightly sealed storage container. Use within 12 months.

Steep 1-2 tbsp of tea blend per 8 fl oz (240 mL) freshly boiled hot water in a heat-safe container, covered, for 5-7 minutes.

Strain infusion through a tea strainer and compost or discard plant material.

Serve and enjoy!

Drink one 8 fl oz serving after a heavy meal.

Gentle
DANDY DETOX TEA

Give the liver a bit of gentle support after the winter season, when signs of congestion or burden show up, or any time you want to give it a bit of nourishment with this blend of herbs. Note: If preferred, use anise (*Pimpinella anisum*) seed in place of licorice root.

Yield: 1⅛ cups dried tea blend

INGREDIENTS

¼ cup dandelion (*Taraxacum officinale*) root

¼ cup dandelion (*Taraxacum officinale*) leaf

¼ cup nettle (*Urtica dioica*) leaf

¼ cup green tea (*Camellia sinensis*) leaf (or additional nettle leaf for a caffeine-free option)

2 tbsp licorice (*Glycyrrhiza glabra*) root

DIRECTIONS

Combine all ingredients and store the blend in a labeled, tightly sealed storage container. Use within 12 months.

Steep 1 tbsp of tea blend per 8 fl oz (240 mL) freshly boiled hot water in a heat-safe container, covered, for 5-10 minutes.

Strain infusion through a tea strainer and compost or discard plant material.

Serve and enjoy!

Drink up to three 8 fl oz servings per day.

GENTLE
digestive tea

A favorite digestive blend adapted from the After Dinner Tea recipe in Herbal Academy's Intermediate Herbal Course.

Yield: One 8 fl oz serving

INGREDIENTS

1 ½ tbsp chamomile (*Matricaria chamomilla*) flower

½ tsp orange (*Citrus* spp.) peel

½ tsp anise (*Pimpinella anisum*) seed

8 fl oz (240 mL) water

DIRECTIONS

Place herbs in a heat-safe container.

Pour freshly boiled hot water over the herbs, cover, and steep for 5-10 minutes.

Strain the infusion through a tea strainer and compost or discard plant material.

Serve and enjoy!

Drink up to four servings per day.

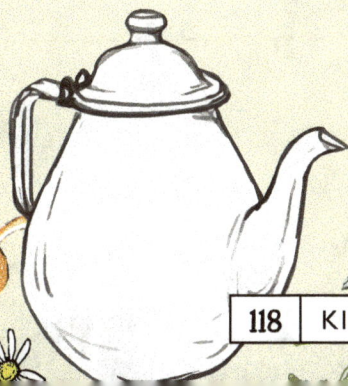

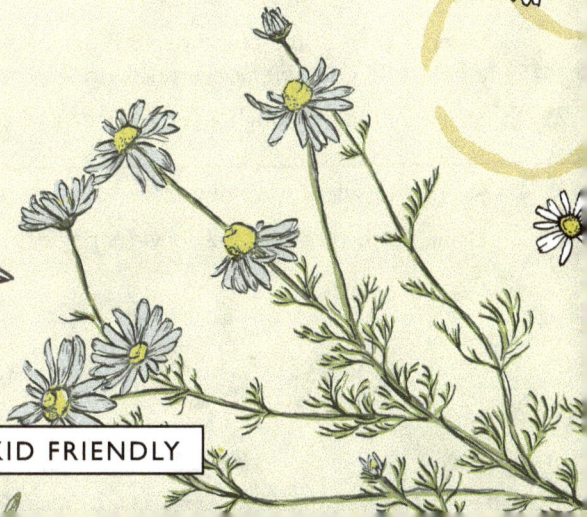

GUT CHECK TEA

The digestive tract is one of the most important body systems in need of regular support for optimal functioning. Not only does it play a role in nutrient absorption and overall wellness, but it is also one of the primary ways the body regulates what is external versus internal. This tea blend is packed with herbs that help to soothe irritated gastrointestinal mucosal lining, stimulate cell regeneration if needed, and strengthen any weak or lax cellular junctions throughout the gastrointestinal tract.

Yield: 2 cups dried tea blend

INGREDIENTS

½ cup calendula (*Calendula officinalis*) flower

½ cup oat (*Avena sativa*) straw

¼ cup chamomile (*Matricaria chamomilla*) flower

¼ cup goldenrod (*Solidago* spp.) aerial parts

¼ cup plantain (*Plantago* spp.) leaf

¼ cup peppermint (*Mentha × piperita*) leaf

DIRECTIONS

Combine all ingredients and store the blend in a labeled, tightly sealed storage container. Use within 12 months.

Steep 1 tbsp of tea blend per 8 fl oz (240 mL) freshly boiled hot water in a heat-safe container, covered, for 5-7 minutes.

Strain infusion through a tea strainer and compost or discard plant material.

Sip hot, or allow to cool and serve over ice.

Drink up to three 8 fl oz servings per day.

Gut Soothing
Herbal Tea

Digestion is the seat of health, and when the system's tissues are inflamed, health will suffer. With its combination of vulnerary, demulcent, carminative, and antispasmodic herbs, this blend will help to support and strengthen the gut lining of the digestive tract, as well as soothe gastrointestinal upset.

Yield: Four 8 fl oz servings

INGREDIENTS

1 tbsp chamomile (*Matricaria chamomilla*) flower

1 tbsp fennel (*Foeniculum vulgare*) seed

1 tbsp marshmallow (*Althaea officinalis*) root

2 tsp calendula (*Calendula officinalis*) flower

1 tsp peppermint (*Mentha* x *piperita*) leaf

32 fl oz (960 mL) water

DIRECTIONS

Place herbs in a heat-safe container.

Pour freshly boiled hot water over the herbs, cover, and steep for 10 minutes.

Strain the infusion through a tea strainer and compost or discard plant material.

Serve and enjoy!

Consume immediately or within 24 hours after straining, if refrigerated.

Drink up to four servings per day.

| KID FRIENDLY

Happy Belly
OVERNIGHT INFUSION

The recipe features marshmallow and calendula, two vulnerary herbs that support gut health and help strengthen intestinal integrity. Marshmallow contains carbohydrates called mucilage that are best extracted in cold water, which is why this recipe has two different infusion steps. Mucilage has a somewhat slimy consistency (this is what helps it coat the stomach lining with supportive goodness), but if the drink is too gooey for you, then try swapping marshmallow root for marshmallow leaf, which is still effective but contains less mucilage so will be less slimy.

Yield: Eight 8 fl oz servings

INGREDIENTS

½ cup marshmallow (*Althaea officinalis*) root or leaf

½ cup calendula (*Calendula officinalis*) aerial parts

¼ cup peppermint (*Mentha* x *piperita*) leaf

64 fl oz (1.9 L) water

DIRECTIONS

Place marshmallow root or leaf in a glass jar.

Pour 32 fl oz (960 mL) of room temperature water over the marshmallow, cover, and steep overnight.

At the same time, place calendula and peppermint in a heat-safe container.

Pour 32 fl oz (960 mL) of just boiled hot water over the herbs, cover, and steep overnight.

Strain both infusions through a tea strainer and compost or discard plant material.

Mix infusions together, serve, and enjoy.

Consume immediately or within 24 hours after straining, if refrigerated.

Drink up to eight servings per day.

HEATHER'S
BUZZY BEE TEA

This mint-family forward tea combines tart, refreshing flavors to make magic in your mouth and bring peace to your digestive system. Vibrant bright green new tips from edible evergreens give it a piney-fresh taste. - Heather Wood Buzzard

Yield: One 8 fl oz serving

INGREDIENTS

1 tsp bee balm (*Monarda fistulosa*) aerial parts

1 tsp lemon balm (*Melissa officinalis*) aerial parts or sumac (*Rhus* spp.) berry

½ tsp peppermint (*Mentha x piperita*) leaf

½ tsp spearmint (*Mentha spicata*) leaf

½ tsp fresh spruce (*Picea* spp.), pine (*Pinus* spp.), or Eastern hemlock (*Tsuga canadensis*) young needles (or another edible evergreen), minced

8 fl oz (240 mL) water

DIRECTIONS

Place herbs in a heat-safe container.

Pour freshly boiled hot water over the herbs, cover, and steep for 10-15 minutes.

Strain the infusion through a tea strainer and compost or discard plant material.

Serve and enjoy!

Drink up to four servings per day.

Lemon Surprise
ICED TEA

Whether you want to cool off, cleanse your palate, or stimulate your appetite, this lemony tea is a flavorful way to do all of the above. Enjoy it sweet or sour—just enjoy it!

Yield: 1⅝ cups dried tea blend

INGREDIENTS

1 cup lemon balm (*Melissa officinalis*) leaf

¼ cup ginger (*Zingiber officinale*) rhizome

¼ cup dried lemon slices, chopped

2 tbsp fennel (*Foeniculum vulgare*) seed

DIRECTIONS

Combine all ingredients and store the blend in a labeled, tightly sealed storage container. Use within 12 months.

Steep 1 tbsp of tea blend per 8 fl oz (240 mL) freshly boiled hot water in a heat-safe container, covered, for 5-10 minutes.

Strain infusion through a tea strainer and compost or discard plant material.

Place in the refrigerator and allow to cool.

Serve over ice and enjoy!

Drink up to three 8 fl oz servings per day.

~MINTY~
Ginger Tea

Mint and ginger pair so well in this digestion-supporting blend. Perfect for an after-dinner drink to help ease gas and bloating, or to aid the body when a stomachache arises. Enjoy this spicy, warming tea with family or friends when the meal is done!

Yield: Approximately three 8 fl oz servings

INGREDIENTS

2-inch piece fresh ginger (*Zingiber officinale*) rhizome, chopped

2 tbsp peppermint (*Mentha × piperita*) or spearmint (*Mentha spicata*) leaf

2 tbsp chamomile (*Matricaria chamomilla*) flower

32 fl oz (960 mL) water

DIRECTIONS

Place ginger in a saucepan with water.

Bring to a boil, cover, then reduce the heat to a simmer.

Simmer for 20 minutes.

Remove from heat, add mint, cover, and steep for 5 minutes.

Add chamomile, cover, and steep for another 5 minutes.

Strain decoction into a heat-safe container using a tea strainer, and compost or discard plant material.

Serve and enjoy!

Consume immediately or within 48 hours after straining, if refrigerated.

Drink up to four servings per day.

KID + PREGNANCY FRIENDLY

SOOTHE *the gut* TEA

This tea blend is perfect for those experiencing systemic issues stemming from intestinal permeability concerns. As a warming, vulnerary digestive infusion, it will support a digestive tract that could use some extra soothing, and with all the aromatic herbs it tastes great, too!
- Shona Richter MacDougall

Yield: 1¼ cups dried tea blend

INGREDIENTS

¼ cup calendula (*Calendula officinalis*) flower

3 tbsp catnip (*Nepeta cataria*) aerial parts

3 tbsp peppermint (*Mentha* x *piperita*) leaf

3 tbsp plantain (*Plantago* spp.) leaf

3 tbsp ginger (*Zingiber officinale*) rhizome

2 tbsp chamomile (*Matricaria chamomilla*) flower

2 tbsp cardamom (*Elettaria cardamomum*) pod, crushed

DIRECTIONS

Combine all ingredients and store the blend in a labeled, tightly sealed storage container. Use within 12 months.

Steep ⅓ cup of tea blend per 32 fl oz (960 mL) freshly boiled hot water in a heat-safe container, covered, for 4 hours or overnight.

Strain infusion through a tea strainer and compost or discard plant material.

Serve and enjoy!

Consume immediately or within 24 hours after straining, if refrigerated.

Drink up to four 8 fl oz servings per day.

KID FRIENDLY

spiced rose
AFTER-DINNER TEA

This warming, carminative tea blend is just the thing if you want the flavor of chai, but are looking for a relaxing option that doesn't contain caffeine.

Yield: Four 8 fl oz servings

INGREDIENTS

1 tbsp wood betony (*Betonica officinalis*) aerial parts

1 tsp rose (*Rosa* spp.) petal

½ tsp ginger (*Zingiber officinale*) rhizome

½ tsp cardamom (*Elettaria cardamomum*) seed

32 fl oz (960 mL) water

DIRECTIONS

Place herbs in a heat-safe container.

Pour freshly boiled hot water over the herbs, cover, and steep for 20 minutes.

Strain the infusion through a tea strainer and compost or discard plant material.

Serve and enjoy!

Consume immediately or within 24 hours after straining, if refrigerated.

Drink up to four servings per day.

| KID FRIENDLY

Sweet
MELISSA

Sip the flavor of high summer with this relaxing, carminative tea blend, named after lemon balm's genus (*Melissa*), which comes from the Greek word for honeybee. Get ready to be transported to a summer garden humming with happy pollinators!

Yield: Four 8 fl oz servings

INGREDIENTS

2½ tsp wood betony (*Betonica officinalis*) aerial parts

2 tsp lemon balm (*Melissa officinalis*) aerial parts

1 tsp lavender (*Lavandula* spp.) flower bud

⅛ tsp stevia (*Stevia rebaudiana*) leaf

32 fl oz (960 mL) water

DIRECTIONS

Place herbs in a heat-safe container.

Pour freshly boiled hot water over the herbs, cover, and steep for 20 minutes.

Strain the infusion through a tea strainer and compost or discard plant material.

Serve and enjoy!

Consume immediately or within 24 hours after straining, if refrigerated.

Drink up to four servings per day.

CA-*mo*-BALM *tea*

This simple formula utilizes three multifaceted herbs to create a powerhouse blend that's also sweet, gentle, and tasty. Calming and uplifting to the nervous system, carminative and soothing to the digestive system, and clearing to the respiratory system, this tea makes a soothing blend for tummy aches, colds, and restlessness at bedtime. This is an especially nice blend for children, but it finds favor with teens and adults as well.
- Jane Metzger

Yield: 1¼ cups dried tea blend

INGREDIENTS

½ cup chamomile (*Matricaria chamomilla*) flower

½ cup lemon balm (*Melissa officinalis*) aerial parts

¼ cup catnip (*Nepeta cataria*) leaf

DIRECTIONS

Combine all ingredients and store the blend in a labeled, tightly sealed storage container. Use within 12 months.

Steep 1 tbsp of tea blend per 8 fl oz (240 mL) freshly boiled hot water in a heat-safe container, covered, for 5-7 minutes.

Strain infusion through a tea strainer and compost or discard plant material.

Serve and enjoy!

Drink up to four 8 fl oz servings per day.

Energize & Uplift

Botanical blends that boost energy,
sharpen mental focus and clarity, put a
delightful pep in our step, invite creativity
and enchantment, offer solace, and support
self love.

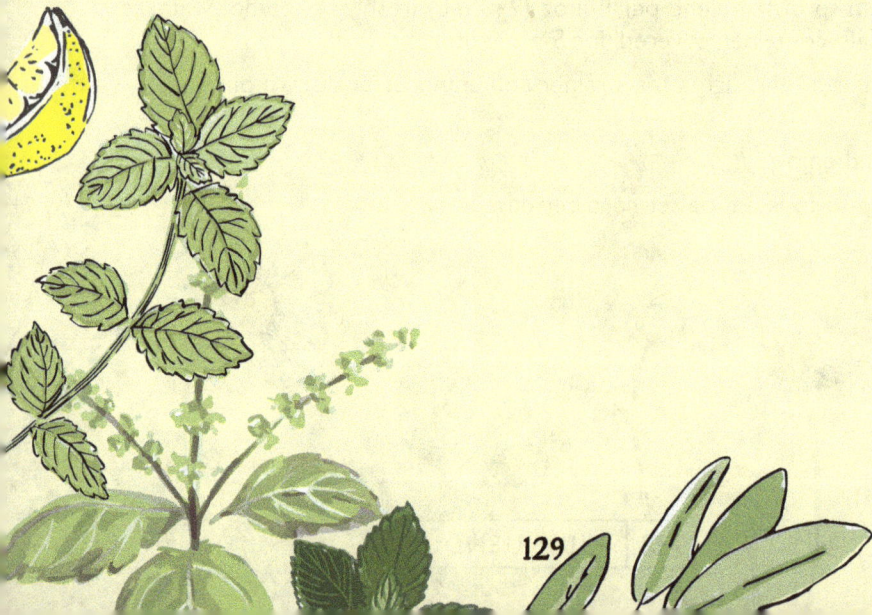

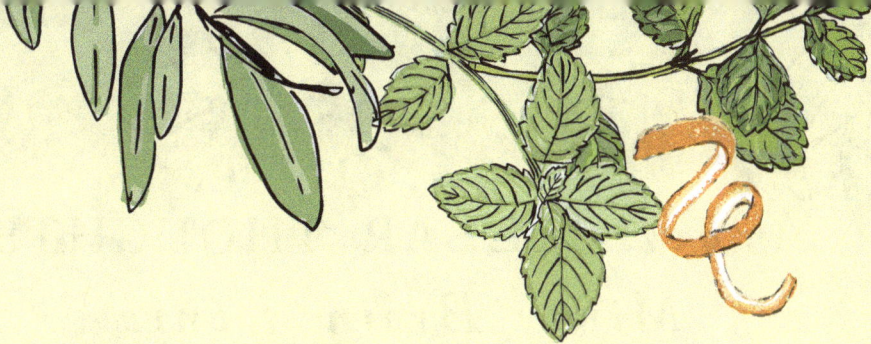

RECIPES:

Amber's CLEAR THOUGHTS
Minty Brain Tonic

Personally, when I need a boost of energy, it's typically because I'm experiencing mental fatigue. This is my go-to cup of afternoon tea for mental clarity and refresh for a productive work session. With its nervous system and cardiovascular system benefits, this blend is sure to support healthy brain function and help you have clarity, focus, and energy in whatever task is ahead! I will often prepare large batches of this blend, store it in the fridge, and pour it over ice when needed—having it easily available for an afternoon pick-me-up is always welcomed when that slowdown kicks in!
- Amber Meyers

Yield: Two 8 fl oz servings

INGREDIENTS

2 tbsp spearmint (*Mentha spicata*) leaf

1 tbsp tulsi (*Ocimum tenuiflorum*) aerial parts

2 tsp sage (*Salvia officinalis*) leaf

2 tsp rosemary (*Salvia rosmarinus*) leaf (optional)

16 fl oz (480 mL) water

DIRECTIONS

Place herbs in a heat-safe container.

Pour freshly boiled hot water over the herbs, cover, and steep for 5-20 minutes.

Strain the infusion through a tea strainer and compost or discard plant material.

Sip hot, or allow to cool and serve over ice, and enjoy!

Drink up to two servings before work or study sessions.

| KID FRIENDLY

BUSY BEE
HERBAL TEA

The perfect tea for those times when you want to hone in on a project and accomplish a lot. Enjoy this tea hot or cold depending on what you're feeling at the present moment, and turn your attention to focus on the task ahead.

Yield: 1⅞ cups dried tea blend

INGREDIENTS

¾ cup lemon balm (*Melissa officinalis*) aerial parts

½ cup gotu kola (*Centella asiatica*) leaf

¼ cup tulsi (*Ocimum tenuiflorum*) aerial parts

¼ cup rose (*Rosa* spp.) petal

2 tbsp peppermint (*Mentha x piperita*) leaf

DIRECTIONS

Combine all ingredients and store the blend in a labeled, tightly sealed storage container. Use within 12 months.

Steep 1 tbsp of tea blend per 8 fl oz (240 mL) freshly boiled hot water in a heat-safe container, covered, for 10-15 minutes.

Strain infusion through a tea strainer and compost or discard plant material.

Serve and enjoy!

Drink up to three 8 fl oz servings per day.

KID FRIENDLY

Hannah's Writing
TEA

As an herbal writer, I need to stay mentally focused and alert while working on projects. I try not to drink much caffeine after noon, but sometimes I need a stronger pick-me-up to make a deadline. I've found that this tea blend provides just enough caffeine to invigorate my senses, while keeping my nervous system balanced and my sleep on track. For kids and if desired in pregnancy, opt for the caffeine-free nettle version.
- Hannah Lasorsa

Yield: One 8 fl oz serving

INGREDIENTS

1 tsp green tea (*Camellia sinensis*) leaf (or nettle (*Urtica dioica*) leaf for a caffeine-free option)

1 tsp peppermint (*Mentha x piperita*) leaf

1 tsp oat (*Avena sativa*) straw

8 fl oz (240 mL) water

DIRECTIONS

Place herbs in a heat-safe container.

Pour freshly boiled hot water over the herbs, cover, and steep for 5 minutes.

Strain the infusion through a tea strainer and compost or discard plant material.

Serve and enjoy!

Drink up to two servings per day.

133 | KID + PREGNANCY FRIENDLY

HEARTWARMING
TEA

A blend of herbs that combine to create a cup of tea that feels like an enlivening hug for the heart. Reach for this blend when you're feeling down and you need the support of your herbal allies.

Yield: One 8 fl oz serving

INGREDIENTS

1 tbsp rose (*Rosa* spp.) petal

1 tsp peppermint (*Mentha* x *piperita*) leaf

½ tsp cinnamon (*Cinnamomum* spp.) bark, crushed

8 fl oz (240 mL) water

DIRECTIONS

Place herbs in a heat-safe container.

Pour freshly boiled hot water over the herbs, cover, and steep for 10-15 minutes.

Strain the infusion through a tea strainer and compost or discard plant material.

Serve and enjoy!

Drink up to four servings per day.

Herbal "Earl Grey" Tea

An herbal twist on the classic tea recipe, this botanically infused "Earl Grey" tea blend can be enjoyed any time of day. Add in a splash of milk and a drizzle of honey, and you've practically got yourself a dessert! For a caffeine-free version, use the raspberry leaf option.

Yield: 1¼ cups dried tea blend

INGREDIENTS

1 cup black tea (*Camellia sinensis*) leaf (or raspberry (*Rubus idaeus*) leaf for a caffeine-free option)

¼ cup violet (*Viola odorata* or *V. sororia*) flower

10-15 drops bergamot (*Citrus x bergamia*) essential oil

DIRECTIONS

Add essential oil drops to a quart sized glass canning jar, rotating the jar so the oil spreads across as much of the bottom and sides of the jar as possible.

Add all plant material to the jar, cap and label, and shake the jar well to mix the herbs together and expose as much of the plant material as possible to the essential oil on the jar.

Set the jar aside to rest for 24-48 hours before making a cup of tea to test the flavor.

If additional flavor is needed, repeat the above steps once more before storing the blend in a labeled, tightly sealed storage container for up to 12 months.

Steep 1-2 tsp of tea blend per 8 fl oz (240 mL) freshly boiled hot water in a heat-safe container, covered, for 5-7 minutes.

Strain infusion through a tea strainer and compost or discard plant material.

Add milk of choice (dairy or non-dairy) and sweeten with honey (or sweetener of choice) to taste, if desired.

Serve and enjoy!

Drink up to two 8 fl oz servings per day.

LAND *of the* FAERIES TEA

Light, enchanting, and mysterious, this tea blend features delicate herbs that soothe, moisten, and strengthen the tissues of the body while cheering the heart and lightening the mind. And if the beauty of this herbal tea blend doesn't transport you to the land of the faeries, the flavor certainly will.

Yield: 2 cups dried tea blend

INGREDIENTS

¾ cup plantain (*Plantago* spp.) leaf

½ cup rose (*Rosa* spp.) petal

½ cup lemon balm (*Melissa officinalis*) aerial parts

¼ cup calendula (*Calendula officinalis*) flower

DIRECTIONS

Combine all ingredients and store the blend in a labeled, tightly sealed storage container. Use within 12 months.

Steep 1 tbsp of tea blend per 8 fl oz (240 mL) freshly boiled hot water in a heat-safe container, covered, for 5-10 minutes.

Strain infusion through a tea strainer and compost or discard plant material.

Sip hot, or allow to cool and serve over ice.

Drink up to three 8 fl oz servings per day.

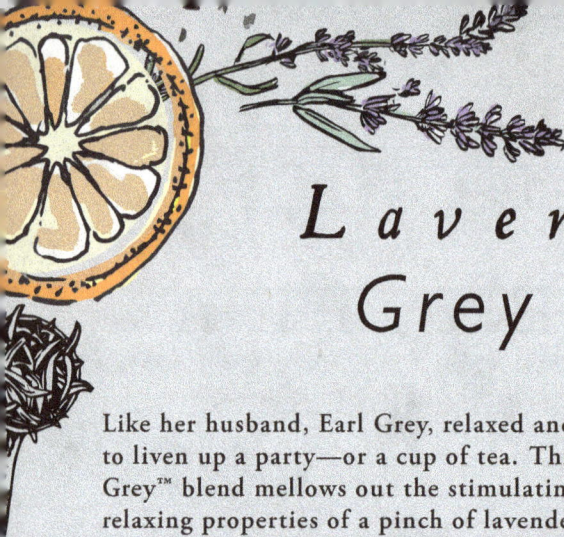

Lavender Grey Tea

Like her husband, Earl Grey, relaxed and refined Lady Grey knows how to liven up a party—or a cup of tea. This twist on the classic Lady Grey™ blend mellows out the stimulating effects of black tea with the relaxing properties of a pinch of lavender while adding an extra pop of citrus flavor. For a caffeine-free version, use the raspberry leaf option.

Yield: 1⅛ cups dried tea blend

INGREDIENTS

1 cup black tea (*Camellia sinensis*) leaf (or raspberry (*Rubus* idaeus) leaf for a caffeine-free option)

1 tbsp lavender (*Lavandula* spp.) flower bud

10-15 drops bergamot (*Citrus* x *bergamia*) essential oil

1 tbsp each lemon and orange slices, chopped

DIRECTIONS

Add essential oil drops to a quart sized glass canning jar, rotating the jar so the oil spreads across as much of the bottom and sides of the jar as possible.

Add all plant material to the jar, cap and label, and shake the jar well to mix the herbs together and expose as much of the plant material as possible to the essential oil on the jar.

Set the jar aside to rest for 24-48 hours before making a cup of tea to test the flavor.

If additional flavor is needed, repeat the above steps once more before storing the blend in a labeled, tightly sealed storage container for up to 12 months.

Steep 1-2 tsp of tea blend per 8 fl oz (240 mL) freshly boiled hot water in a heat-safe container, covered, for 5-10 minutes.

Strain infusion through a tea strainer and compost or discard plant material.

Sweeten with honey (or sweetener of choice) to taste, if desired.

Serve and enjoy!

Drink up to two 8 fl oz servings per day.

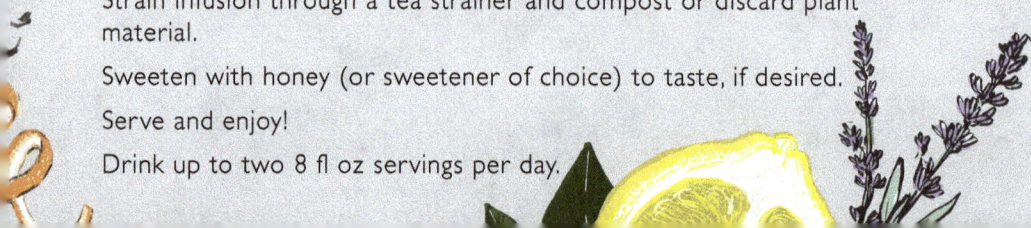

LION'S MANE
MATCHA TEA

This energizing beverage is warm and comforting and supports mental calm and focus. It's a wonderful substitute for your morning coffee and makes a terrific addition to study sessions or any other activity that calls for focus and mental work. For a caffeine-free version, use powdered nettle leaf in place of matcha powder.

Yield: One 8 fl oz serving

INGREDIENTS

¼-½ tsp lion's mane (*Hericium erinaceus*) mushroom extract powder

½ tsp matcha (*Camellia sinensis*) leaf powder (or nettle (*Urtica dioica*) leaf, powdered, for a caffeine-free option)

8 fl oz (240 mL) water (or milk of choice (dairy or non-dairy))

Honey (or sweetener of choice) to taste (optional)

DIRECTIONS

Place powdered herbs in a heat-safe mug.

Pour freshly boiled hot water over the herbs until the mug is about ¼ full. (If you prefer a latte-style matcha, substitute warmed milk instead of water.)

Use a whisk or fork to stir briskly for 30 seconds.

Add the remainder of the hot water (or milk, if using).

Add sweetener to taste, if desired.

Drink up to two servings per day.

PEP *in your* STEP
MEMORY TEA

This blend highlights rosemary and is lovely for recalling memories, a train of thought, or information during journaling or the writing process. Tulsi and orange peel harmonize with rosemary for an earthy flavor while mint and sage wake up the senses, offering focus and inspiration.

Yield: 1¾ cups dried tea blend

INGREDIENTS

½ cup mint (*Mentha* spp.) leaf

½ cup tulsi (*Ocimum tenuiflorum*) aerial parts

¼ cup rosemary (*Salvia rosmarinus*) leaf

¼ cup sage (*Salvia officinalis*) leaf

¼ cup orange (*Citrus* spp.) peel

DIRECTIONS

Combine all ingredients and store the blend in a labeled, tightly sealed storage container. Use within 12 months.

Steep 2 tsp of tea blend per 8 fl oz (240 mL) freshly boiled hot water in a heat-safe container, covered, for 10-15 minutes.

Strain infusion through a tea strainer and compost or discard plant material.

Serve and enjoy!

Drink up to three 8 fl oz servings per day.

| KID FRIENDLY

REMEMBRANCE
t e a

Give your memory a boost with this caffeine-rich, aromatic tea that will not only give you a bit of energy but will also increase blood flow to your brain, thus providing it with more nourishment so you are alert and better able to think clearly. For kids, opt for the caffeine-free raspberry leaf version.

Yield: Two 8 fl oz servings

INGREDIENTS

1 tbsp black tea (*Camellia sinensis*) leaf (or raspberry (*Rubus idaeus*) leaf for a caffeine-free option)

2 tsp rosemary (*Salvia rosmarinus*) leaf

1 tsp orange (*Citrus* spp.) peel

16 fl oz (480 mL) water

Milk of choice (dairy or non-dairy) (optional)

Honey (or sweetener of choice) to taste (optional)

DIRECTIONS

Place herbs in a heat-safe container.

Pour freshly boiled hot water over the herbs, cover, and steep for 7-8 minutes.

Strain the infusion through a tea strainer and compost or discard plant material.

Add milk and honey, if desired.

Serve and enjoy!

Drink up to six servings per day.

Rosemary Gladstar's *Uplifting Tea*

In an interview in celebration of Herbalist's Day, Rosemary shared this recipe with the Herbal Academy community, and it's become a happy favorite! Give this easily adaptable formula from a beloved herbalist a try anytime you need a bit more pep in your step! Packed with uplifting nervines, this tasty tea is sure to give your mood a boost when you need it.

Yield: 1¼ cups dried tea blend

INGREDIENTS

¼ cup hawthorn (*Crataegus* spp.) leaf, flower, and berry

¼ cup lemon balm (*Melissa officinalis*) aerial parts, freshly dried

¼ cup oat (*Avena sativa*) milky seed

¼ cup St. John's wort (*Hypericum perforatum*) aerial parts

¼ cup rose (*Rosa* spp.) petal

1 butterfly pea (*Clitoria ternatea*) flower per cup (optional)

DIRECTIONS

Combine all ingredients, except optional botanicals, and store the blend in a labeled, tightly sealed storage container. Use within 12 months.

Steep 1 tbsp of tea blend, making sure 1 butterfly pea flower is added (if using), per 8 fl oz (240 mL) freshly boiled hot water in a heat-safe container, covered, for 20-30 minutes.

Strain infusion through a tea strainer and compost or discard plant material.

Sweeten with a pinch of stevia or a spoonful of honey, if desired.

Serve and enjoy!

Drink up to four 8 fl oz servings per day.

SWEETBRIAR
- solace -

This comforting cup of tea is perfect on cold, rainy days when you could use a little hug from your herbal allies. Particularly lovely with sweetbriar (*Rosa rugosa*) petals, but any aromatic rose will do!
- Lisa Olson

Yield: Four 8 fl oz servings

INGREDIENTS

1 tbsp peppermint (*Mentha x piperita*) leaf

1 tbsp rose (*Rosa* spp.) petal

2 tsp licorice (*Glycyrrhiza glabra*) root

32 fl oz (960 mL) water

DIRECTIONS

Place herbs in a heat-safe container.

Pour freshly boiled hot water over the herbs, cover, and steep for 20 minutes.

Strain the infusion through a tea strainer and compost or discard plant material.

Consume immediately or within 24 hours after straining, if refrigerated.

Drink up to four servings per day.

Tulsi Love Potion

A relaxing sweet, spicy, and floral tea blend that can help to foster feelings of self love. Drink this tea when you need more self care, to ease the pain of grief, or share it with a friend to awaken the heart center and help the good vibes to flow!
- Alison Birks

Yield: One 12 fl oz serving

INGREDIENTS

2 tsp tulsi (*Ocimum tenuiflorum*) aerial parts

1 tsp cardamom (*Elettaria cardamomum*) pod, crushed

1 tsp rose (*Rosa* spp.) petal

½ tsp crystallized ginger (*Zingiber officinale*) rhizome, minced

12 fl oz (360 mL) water

DIRECTIONS

Place herbs and crystallized ginger in a heat-safe container.

Pour freshly boiled hot water over the herbs, cover, and steep for 15 minutes.

Strain the infusion through a tea strainer and compost or discard plant material.

Serve and enjoy!

Drink up to three servings per day.

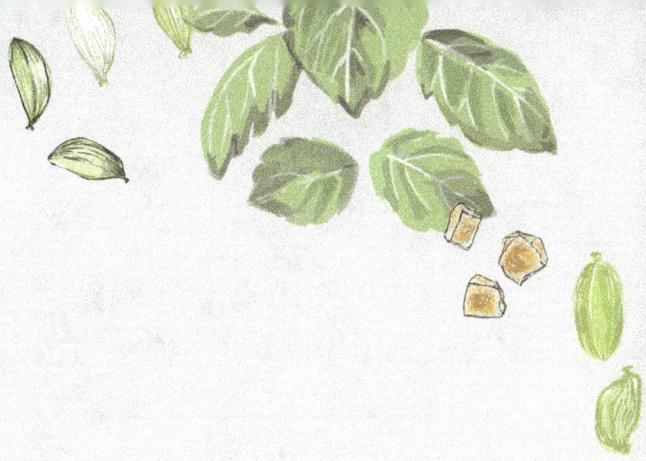

Tea is one of the most enjoyable daily rituals that can accompany your herbal practice, and there's a time-tested, delicious tea blend for nearly every mood or need.

HERBAL ACADEMY

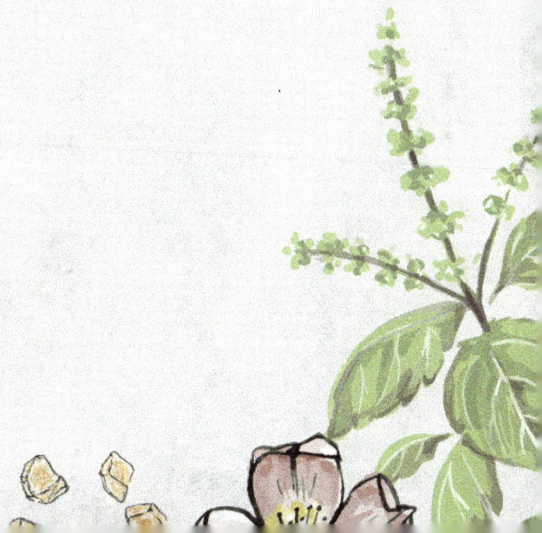

Generate & Eliminate

Botanical blends that address common complaints in the urinary and reproductive systems, easing uncomfortable symptoms, and ensuring smooth function.

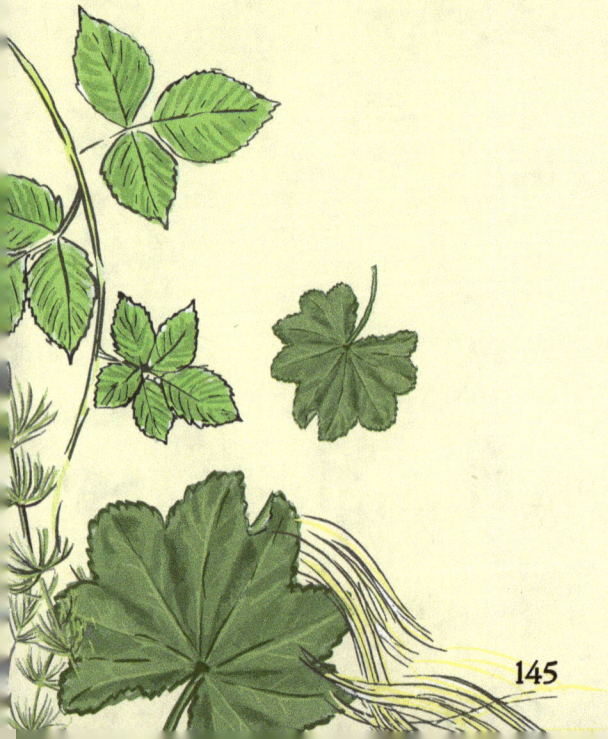

RECIPES:

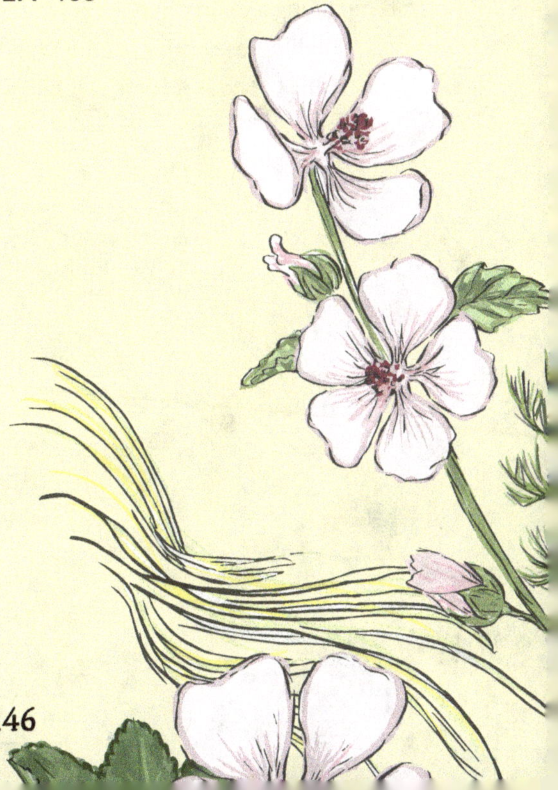

Juicy Bits Tea

For those moving through the menopause transition, tissue can become dry and uncomfortable. This blend is curated to get things moistened, with shatavari leading the blend with its nourishing and moistening strengths. Paired with some top demulcents, this blend is sure to reduce dryness.

Yield: 2 cups dried tea blend

INGREDIENTS

1 cup shatavari (*Asparagus racemosus*) root, powdered

½ cup violet (*Viola odorata* or *V. sororia*) leaf

½ cup marshmallow (*Althaea officinalis*) root, powdered

DIRECTIONS

Combine all ingredients and store the blend in a labeled, tightly sealed storage container. Use within 12 months.

Steep 2 tbsp of tea blend per 8 fl oz (240 mL) freshly boiled hot water in a heat-safe container, covered, for 10-15 minutes.

Strain infusion through a tea strainer and compost or discard plant material.

Sip hot, or allow to cool and serve over ice.

Drink up to four 8 fl oz servings per day.

Lady's Mint Tea

Sip this raspberry leaf tea with lady's mantle to regenerate your body and mind. Choose from iron and vitamin A-rich peppermint or spearmint to support your nutrition and add a dynamic aroma and flavor to the tea.

Yield: 1⅝ cups dried tea blend

INGREDIENTS

½ cup raspberry (*Rubus idaeus*) leaf

½ cup lady's mantle (*Alchemilla vulgaris*) leaf

¼ cup nettle (*Urtica dioica*) leaf

¼ cup peppermint (*Mentha x piperita*) or spearmint (*Mentha spicata*) leaf

2 tbsp rose (*Rosa* spp.) petal

DIRECTIONS

Combine all ingredients and store the blend in a labeled, tightly sealed storage container. Use within 12 months.

Steep ¼ cup of tea blend per 32 fl oz (960 mL) freshly boiled hot water in a heat-safe container, covered, for 4 hours to overnight.

Strain infusion through a tea strainer and compost or discard plant material.

Rewarm if desired, or allow to cool and serve over ice, and enjoy!

Consume immediately or within 24 hours after straining, if refrigerated.

Drink up to four 8 fl oz servings per day.

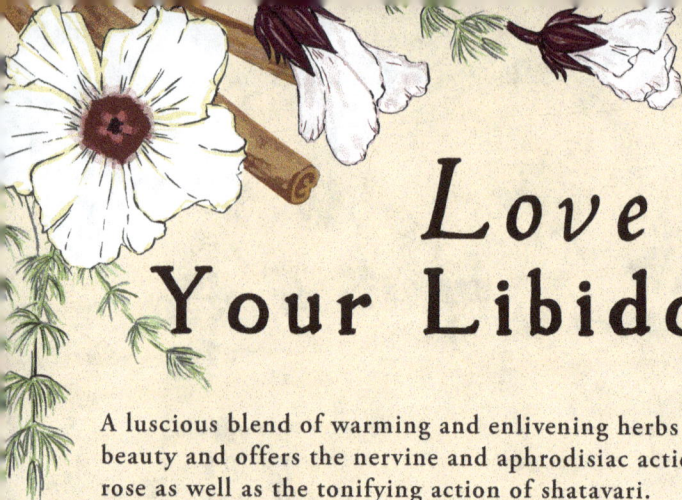

Love Your Libido Tea

A luscious blend of warming and enlivening herbs enchants with its beauty and offers the nervine and aphrodisiac action of damiana and rose as well as the tonifying action of shatavari.

Yield: 1 cup dried tea blend

INGREDIENTS

¼ cup damiana (*Turnera diffusa*) aerial parts

¼ cup hibiscus (*Hibiscus sabdariffa*) calyx

3 tbsp cinnamon (*Cinnamomum* spp.) bark, crushed

2 tbsp rose (*Rosa* spp.) petal

2 tbsp shatavari (*Asparagus racemosus*) root, powdered

DIRECTIONS

Combine all ingredients and store the blend in a labeled, tightly sealed storage container. Use within 12 months.

Steep 1 tbsp of tea blend per 8 fl oz (240 mL) freshly boiled hot water in a heat-safe container, covered, for 15 minutes.

Strain infusion through a tea strainer and compost or discard plant material.

Serve and enjoy!

Drink up to four 8 fl oz servings per day.

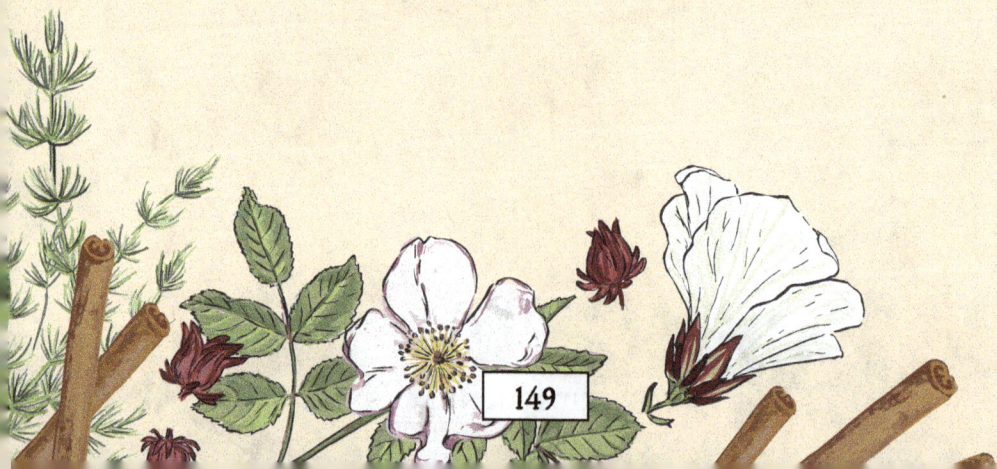

MOON CYCLE TEA

Painful period cramps may be common, but that doesn't mean they can't be helped. This botanical blend will need a few cycles to work its magic, but might be just the thing to help balance the menstrual cycle and ease cramping. Start drinking this tea 5 days prior to the start of menstruation and continue to drink it throughout your moon time.

Yield: Two 8 fl oz servings

INGREDIENTS

2 tsp lady's mantle (*Alchemilla vulgaris*) leaf

1 tsp raspberry (*Rubus idaeus*) leaf

1 tsp hibiscus (*Hibiscus sabdariffa*) calyx

1 tsp yarrow (*Achillea millefolium*) aerial parts

16 fl oz (480 mL) water

DIRECTIONS

Place herbs in a heat-safe container.

Pour freshly boiled hot water over the herbs, cover, and steep for 10 minutes.

Strain the infusion through a tea strainer and compost or discard plant material.

Serve and enjoy!

Drink up to two servings per day.

Prostate
Support Tea

Show your prostate a little support with this botanical brew. The prostate is a lowkey gland until it becomes inflamed, and then it can get one's attention rather quickly. Thankfully, there are herbs that help ease inflammation, deter microbes, tone tissues, and add moisture to support the prostate and urinary tract. Because this includes horsetail (which can deplete thiamine over time), it is meant to be consumed on a short-term basis.

Yield: Approximately four 8 fl oz servings

INGREDIENTS

2 tbsp nettle (*Urtica dioica*) root

½ tbsp horsetail (*Equisetum arvense*) leaf

½ tbsp bee balm (*Monarda fistulosa* or *M. didyma*) aerial parts

½ tbsp corn (*Zea mays*) pistil (silk)

½ tbsp plantain (*Plantago* spp.) leaf

½ tbsp goldenrod (*Solidago* spp.) aerial parts

40 fl oz (720 mL) water

DIRECTIONS

Place nettle root and horsetail in a saucepan with water.

Bring to a boil, cover, then reduce the heat to a simmer.

Simmer for 20 minutes.

Remove from heat, add remaining herbs, cover, and steep for 15-30 minutes.

Strain decoction into a heat-safe container using a tea strainer, and compost or discard plant material.

Serve and enjoy!

Consume immediately or within 48 hours after straining, if refrigerated.

Drink up to four 8 fl oz servings per day.

REPRODUCTIVE
renewal

This soothing infusion is crafted to promote urinary and reproductive wellness and combines the supportive properties of several herbs with cranberry to help reduce inflammation and tighten and tone the urinary and reproductive system tissues. Because this includes uva ursi (which can have a hepatotoxic effect when used long term) and horsetail (which can deplete thiamine over time), it is meant to be consumed on a short-term basis.

Yield: 1½ cups dried tea blend

INGREDIENTS

¼ cup uva ursi (*Arctostaphylos uva-ursi*) leaf

¼ cup horsetail (*Equisetum arvense*) leaf

¼ cup calendula (*Calendula officinalis*) flower

¼ cup corn (*Zea mays*) pistil (silk)

¼ cup yarrow (*Achillea millefolium*) aerial parts

¼ cup dried cranberries, unsweetened, chopped

DIRECTIONS

Combine all ingredients and store the blend in a labeled, tightly sealed storage container. Use within 12 months.

Steep 1 tbsp of tea blend per 8 fl oz (240 mL) freshly boiled hot water in a heat-safe container, covered, for 15 minutes.

Strain infusion through a tea strainer and compost or discard plant material.

Serve and enjoy!

Drink up to two 8 fl oz servings per day.

UT...OH, NO TEA

This tea blend is intended to soothe and support the bladder and surrounding tissues when microbial overgrowth is suspected, helping to ease pain and inflammation, moisten tissues, and increase urine production to flush microbes out! Because this includes uva ursi (which can have a hepatotoxic effect when used long term), it is meant to be consumed on a short-term basis.

Yield: Four 8 fl oz servings

INGREDIENTS

¼ cup dried cranberries, unsweetened, chopped

4 tsp uva ursi (*Arctostaphylos uva-ursi*) leaf

2 tsp meadowsweet (*Filipendula ulmaria*) aerial parts

2 tsp corn (*Zea mays*) pistil (silk)

2 tsp cramp bark (*Viburnum opulus*) bark

2 tsp marshmallow (*Althaea officinalis*) root

½ tsp cinnamon (*Cinnamomum* spp.) bark, crushed

32 fl oz (960 mL) water

DIRECTIONS

Place herbs in a heat-safe container.

Pour freshly boiled hot water over the herbs, cover, and steep for 10-15 minutes.

Strain the infusion through a tea strainer and compost or discard plant material.

Serve and enjoy!

Consume immediately or within 24 hours after straining, if refrigerated.

Drink four servings per day.

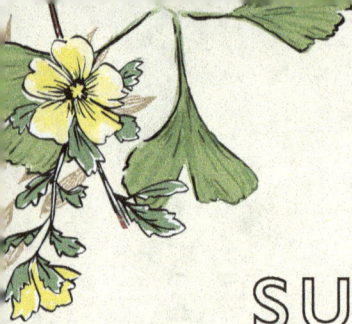

WOMEN
SUPPORT TEA

This recipe yields a strong tea and is blended for women who need herbal allies to support, nourish, and moisten in whichever stage of life. This recipe is based on women's unique needs and is blended using a planetary approach to tea formulation to boost *yin* and *qi*, making it a perfect blend for those feeling dryness and fatigue. While I typically formulate by weight, I have converted measurements to volume for this recipe—hence the specific measurements!
- Holly Hutton

Yield: Two 8 fl oz servings

INGREDIENTS

5 tbsp tulsi (*Ocimum tenuiflorum*) aerial parts

4½ tbsp damiana (*Turnera diffusa*) aerial parts

4½ tbsp oat (*Avena sativa*) straw

2¼ tbsp ginkgo (*Ginkgo biloba*) leaf

1½ tbsp rose (*Rosa* spp.) hip

1¼ tbsp wild yam (*Dioscorea villosa*) root

1 tbsp cardamom (*Elettaria cardamomum*) pod, crushed

2½ tsp shatavari (*Asparagus racemosus*) root

2½ tsp muira puama (*Croton echioides*) root

2 tsp ginger (*Zingiber officinale*) rhizome

1½ tsp ashwagandha (*Withania somnifera*) root

16 fl oz (480 mL) water

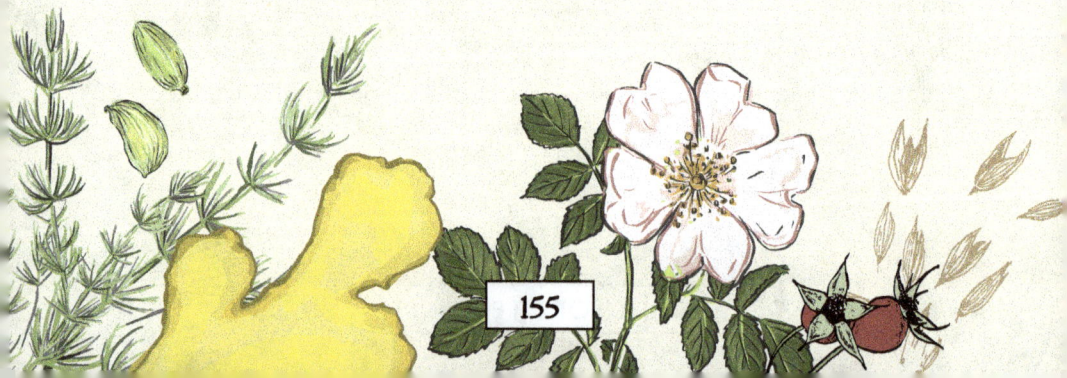

DIRECTIONS

Place herbs in a heat-safe container.

Pour freshly boiled hot water over the herbs, cover, and steep for 10-15 minutes.

Strain the infusion through a tea strainer and compost or discard plant material.

Serve and enjoy!

Drink two 8 fl oz servings per day.

Nourish & Strengthen

Botanical blends that offer adaptogens to support the body's stress response, antioxidants to optimize the cardiovascular system, minerals to strengthen the bones, and nourishing nutrients for tip-top function throughout the body.

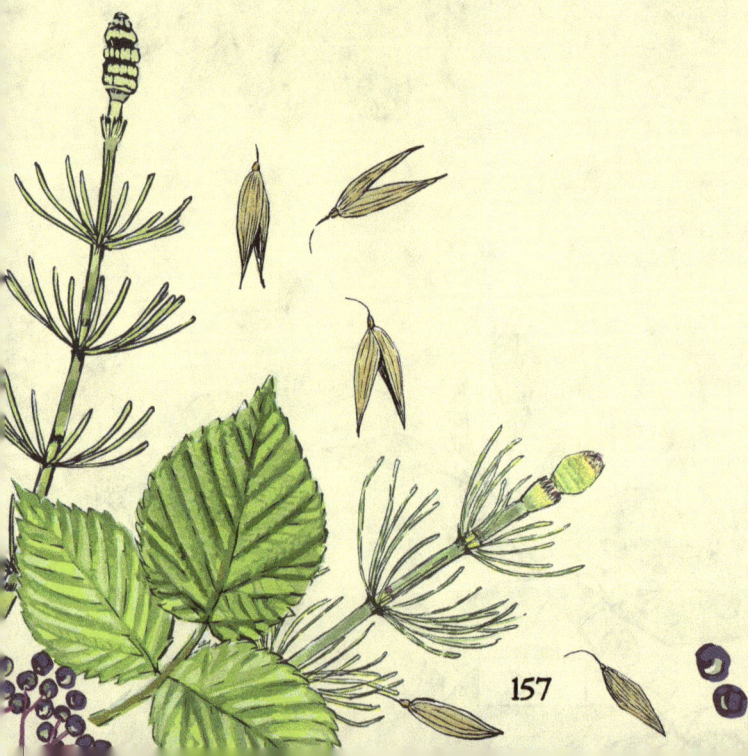

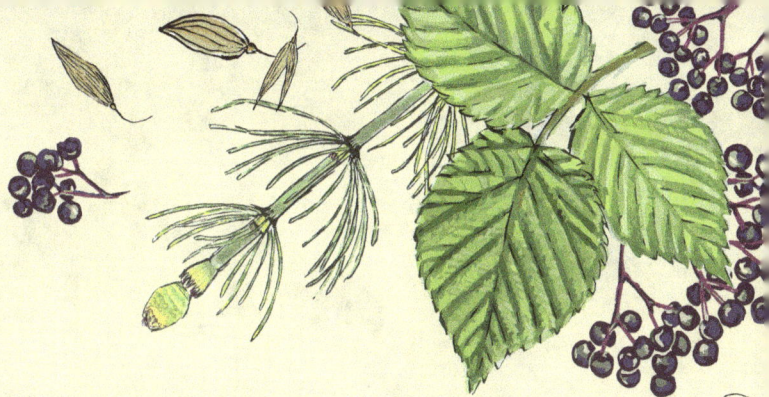

berry spicy FLORAL TEA

What happens when you combine sweet berries, warming spices, and fragrant flowers together? A beautiful and tasty tea blend that's filled with antioxidants, immune support, adaptogen and astringent properties, and so much more—that's what!

Yield: One 12 fl oz serving

INGREDIENTS

I tsp elder (*Sambucus nigra* or *S. canadensis*) berry

I tsp tulsi (*Ocimum tenuiflorum*) aerial parts

I tsp calendula (*Calendula officinalis*) flower

I tsp rose (*Rosa* spp.) petal

I tsp cinnamon (*Cinnamomum* spp.) bark, crushed (or ½ cinnamon stick)

½ tsp ginger (*Zingiber officinale*) rhizome (or 3-4 thin fresh ginger slices)

12 fl oz (360 mL) water

Honey (or sweetener of choice) to taste (optional)

DIRECTIONS

Place herbs in a heat-safe container.

Pour freshly boiled hot water over the herbs, cover, and steep for 15-30 minutes.

Strain the infusion through a tea strainer and compost or discard plant material.

Sweeten with honey, if desired.

Serve and enjoy!

Drink up to three servings per day.

BERRY
blessings

Fill your cup full of the phenolic offerings in this blend of berries and friends. These bright fruits will make a colorful and fruit-forward cup of herbal tea, sure to nourish the mind and the cardiovascular system.

Yield: Approximately three 8 fl oz servings

INGREDIENTS

½ cup fresh blueberries

1 tbsp hawthorn (*Crataegus* spp.) berry

2 tsp elder (*Sambucus nigra* or *S. canadensis*) berry

2 tsp rose (*Rosa* spp.) hip

1 tsp orange (*Citrus* spp.) peel

32 fl oz (960 mL) water

Honey (or sweetener of choice) to taste (optional)

DIRECTIONS

Place herbs and fruit in a saucepan with water.

Bring to a boil, cover, then reduce the heat to a simmer.

Simmer for 20 minutes.

Remove from heat, strain decoction into a heat-safe container using a tea strainer, and compost or discard plant material.

Sweeten with honey, if desired.

Serve and enjoy!

Drink up to three servings per day.

KID FRIENDLY

bone–strengthening
HERBAL INFUSION

This nutrient-rich herbal infusion is packed full of vitamins and minerals from some of our superstar herbal allies, and can be consumed for up to 6 weeks after a break or injury. To support and strengthen overall bone health, substitute red clover for the horsetail, as horsetail may deplete thiamine over time.

Yield: 1½ cups dried tea blend

INGREDIENTS

¼ cup + 2 tbsp rose (*Rosa* spp.) hip

¼ cup lemon balm (*Melissa officinalis*) aerial parts

¼ cup nettle (*Urtica dioica*) leaf

¼ cup oat (*Avena sativa*) straw

¼ cup raspberry (*Rubus idaeus*) leaf

2 tbsp horsetail (*Equisetum arvense*) leaf

DIRECTIONS

Combine all ingredients and store the blend in a labeled, tightly sealed storage container. Use within 12 months.

Steep 3 tbsp of tea blend per 24 fl oz (240 mL) freshly boiled hot water in a heat-safe container, cover, and steep for 1-4 hours or overnight.

Strain infusion through a tea strainer and compost or discard plant material.

Rewarm if desired, serve and enjoy!

Consume immediately or within 24 hours after straining, if refrigerated.

Drink up to three 8 fl oz servings per day.

Calcium + Vitamin C
INFUSION

A blend of nutrient-dense herbs that are perfect for growing children or those who need a bit more calcium and vitamin C in their diets. This tea blend is a tasty way to add needed vitamins and minerals for a healthy body and to pack in a bit more nutrition into your day.

Yield: Four 8 fl oz servings

INGREDIENTS

3 tbsp violet (*Viola odorata* or *V. sororia*) leaf

2 tbsp lemon balm (*Melissa officinalis*) aerial parts

2 tbsp oat (*Avena sativa*) straw

1 tbsp nettle (*Urtica dioica*) leaf

1 tbsp raspberry (*Rubus idaeus*) leaf

½ tbsp cinnamon (*Cinnamomum* spp.) bark, crushed

32 fl oz (960 mL) water

DIRECTIONS

Place herbs in a heat-safe container.

Pour freshly boiled hot water over the herbs, cover, and steep for 1-4 hours or overnight.

Strain the infusion through a tea strainer and compost or discard plant material.

Rewarm if desired, or allow to cool and serve over ice.

Consume immediately or within 24 hours after straining, if refrigerated.

Drink up to four servings per day.

ELEMENTAL BOOST
infusion blend

Go back to the basics with this nutrient-rich infusion blend. Packed with herbs high in minerals, this formula is great for everyday use to support your entire body with some of the minerals it needs to function properly.

Yield: 2¼ cups dried tea blend

INGREDIENTS

½ cup red clover (*Trifolium pratense*) flower

½ cup nettle (*Urtica dioica*) leaf

½ cup dandelion (*Taraxacum officinale*) leaf

½ cup violet (*Viola odorata* or *V. sororia*) aerial parts

8 star anise (*Illicium verum*) seed pods

DIRECTIONS

Combine all ingredients and store the blend in a labeled, tightly sealed storage container. Use within 12 months.

Steep ¼ cup of tea blend, making sure at least one star anise seed pod is included, per 32 fl oz (960 mL) freshly boiled hot water in a heat-safe container, covered, for 4 hours to overnight.

Strain infusion through a tea strainer and compost or discard plant material.

Rewarm if desired, or allow to cool and serve over ice.

Consume immediately or within 24 hours after straining, if refrigerated.

Drink up to four 8 fl oz servings per day.

Green Goddess Tea

Packed with antioxidants, flavonoids, vitamins, minerals, and volatile oils, Green Goddess Tea is good for you from head to toe! With a minty, refreshing flavor, this tea is so yummy and beneficial, it can be enjoyed on a daily basis. For a non-caffeinated option, simply omit the green tea.

Yield: 1¼ cups dried tea blend

INGREDIENTS

½ cup spearmint (*Mentha spicata*) leaf

¼ cup green tea (*Camellia sinensis*) leaf

¼ cup tulsi (*Ocimum tenuiflorum*) aerial parts

2 tbsp nettle (*Urtica dioica*) leaf

1 tbsp rose (*Rosa* spp.) petal

1 tbsp oat (*Avena sativa*) milky seed

DIRECTIONS

Combine all ingredients and store the blend in a labeled, tightly sealed storage container. Use within 12 months.

Steep 1 tbsp of tea blend per 8 fl oz (240 mL) freshly boiled hot water in a heat-safe container, covered, for 3-5 minutes.

Strain infusion through a tea strainer and compost or discard plant material.

Sip hot, or allow to cool and serve over ice with 2-3 fresh spearmint leaves.

Drink up to three 8 fl oz servings per day.

HEART BEETS
TEA BLEND

Fresh fruit and veggies can be a lovely addition to tea blends! This tea is packed with antioxidants that support the health of the entire cardiovascular system, and it makes for a wildly vivid purple-pink drink, too.

Yield: Two 8 fl oz servings

INGREDIENTS

1 handful fresh blackberries

3 fresh beetroot slices

3 fresh blood orange slices

1 tbsp rose (*Rosa* spp.) petal

2 tbsp hawthorn (*Crataegus* spp.) berry

16 fl oz (480 mL) water

DIRECTIONS

Place herbs and fruit in a heat-safe container.

Pour freshly boiled hot water over the herbs and fruit, cover, and steep for 10-15 minutes.

Strain the infusion through a tea strainer and compost or discard plant material.

Serve and enjoy!

Drink up to four servings per day.

heart-strengthening
ROSE TEA

This tea blend is a great one to sip a cup at a time throughout the day for several weeks when you feel your heart could use some nourishment and strength. You can make a large teapot full of it in the morning, making it easy to refill your cup again and again throughout the day.

Yield: 2 cups dried tea blend

INGREDIENTS

1 cup nettle (*Urtica dioica*) leaf

½ cup rose (*Rosa* spp.) petal

½ cup red rooibos (*Aspalathus linearis*) leaf

DIRECTIONS

Combine all ingredients and store the blend in a labeled, tightly sealed storage container. Use within 12 months.

Steep 1 tbsp of tea blend per 8 fl oz (240 mL) freshly boiled hot water in a heat-safe container, covered, for 10 minutes.

Strain infusion through a tea strainer and compost or discard plant material.

Add milk and honey, if desired.

Serve and enjoy!

Drink up to four 8 fl oz servings per day.

HERBAL ACADEMY'S
Nourishing Weedy Tea

Weeds that nourish? Why, yes! Put those nutrient-rich plants to work by infusing them in water and sipping throughout the day to strengthen the body. This blend was one of Herbal Academy's first tea blends shared locally, lovingly packaged up and supplied to vendors!

Yield: Four 8 fl oz servings

INGREDIENTS

¼ cup nettle (*Urtica dioica*) leaf

¼ cup peppermint (*Mentha x piperita*) leaf

¼ cup dandelion (*Taraxacum officinale*) leaf

¼ cup red clover (*Trifolium pratense*) aerial parts

32 fl oz (960 mL) water

DIRECTIONS

Place herbs in a heat-safe container.

Pour freshly boiled hot water over the herbs, cover, and steep for 20 minutes to 4 hours or overnight.

Strain the infusion through a tea strainer and compost or discard plant material.

Rewarm if desired, serve, and enjoy!

Consume immediately or within 24 hours after straining, if refrigerated.

Drink up to four servings per day.

Hibiscus Rose
ICED TEA

This colorful tea is packed with vitamin C and antioxidants and is a great way to support your immunity during the warmer months of the year. Sip a glass or two of this refreshing tea on a warm summer's day, at a garden party with friends, or at a family gathering where a light, refreshing beverage is preferred.

Yield: 1⅞ cups dried tea blend

INGREDIENTS

1 cup hibiscus (*Hibiscus sabdariffa*) calyx

½ cup rose (*Rosa* spp.) petal

¼ cup orange (*Citrus* spp.) peel

2 tbsp ginger (*Zingiber officinale*) rhizome

DIRECTIONS

Combine all ingredients and store the blend in a labeled, tightly sealed storage container. Use within 12 months.

Steep 1 tbsp of tea blend per 8 fl oz (240 mL) freshly boiled hot water in a heat-safe container, covered, for 30 minutes.

Strain infusion through a tea strainer and compost or discard plant material.

Place in the refrigerator and allow to cool.

Serve over ice with a fresh orange round (if desired) and enjoy!

Drink up to three 8 fl oz servings per day.

HIGH-C
hibiscus tea

A sour blend of vitamin C-rich herbs and berries, capable of boosting nutrition while packing a flavorful punch. Whether you're looking to enhance your immune system or promote overall well being, this is a go-to recipe. This sour tea is enjoyable on its own, over ice, or sweetened up with a little honey.

Yield: 1⅜ cups dried tea blend

INGREDIENTS

¼ cup + 2 tbsp hibiscus (*Hibiscus sabdariffa*) calyx

¼ cup + 2 tbsp rose (*Rosa* spp.) hip

¼ cup acerola (*Malpighia* spp.) berry

¼ cup raspberry (*Rubus idaeus*) leaf

2 tbsp lemon (*Citrus* x *limon*) peel

DIRECTIONS

Combine all ingredients and store the blend in a labeled, tightly sealed storage container. Use within 12 months.

Steep 1 tbsp of tea blend per 8 fl oz (240 mL) freshly boiled hot water in a heat-safe container, covered, for 15-20 minutes.

Strain infusion through a tea strainer and compost or discard plant material.

Add honey, if desired.

Serve and enjoy!

Drink up to four 8 fl oz servings per day.

Nutritive Nettle & Tree Tea

Don't let the sting of nettle or the prickly thorns of hawthorn dissuade you from harvesting these nourishing botanicals! This blend will provide a nutritive boost and a tasty cup of tea sure to nourish from the inside out.

Yield: One 8 fl oz serving

INGREDIENTS

1 tbsp nettle (*Urtica dioica*) leaf

1 tsp linden (*Tilia* spp.) flower and bract

1 tsp hawthorn (*Crataegus* spp.) berry, leaf, and/or flower

8 fl oz (240 mL) water

DIRECTIONS

Place herbs in a heat-safe container.

Pour freshly boiled hot water over the herbs, cover, and steep for 15-20 minutes.

Strain the infusion through a tea strainer and compost or discard plant material.

Serve and enjoy!

Drink up to four servings per day.

Overnight
TRIPLE HAWTHORN
infusion

This magical three parts blend of hawthorn is sure to calm the mind and nourish the heart, as it contains inflammation-reducing flavonoids and nervous system-supporting triterpenes. So drink up! Hawthorn's heart-healthy benefits await you.

Yield: One 16 fl oz serving

INGREDIENTS

1 tbsp hawthorn (*Crataegus* spp.) leaf

1 tbsp hawthorn (*Crataegus* spp.) flower

1 tbsp hawthorn (*Crataegus* spp.) berry

16 fl oz (480 mL) water

DIRECTIONS

Place herbs in a heat-safe container.

Pour freshly boiled hot water over the herbs, cover, and steep overnight.

Strain the infusion through a tea strainer and compost or discard plant material.

Rewarm if desired, serve, and enjoy!

Drink up to two servings per day.

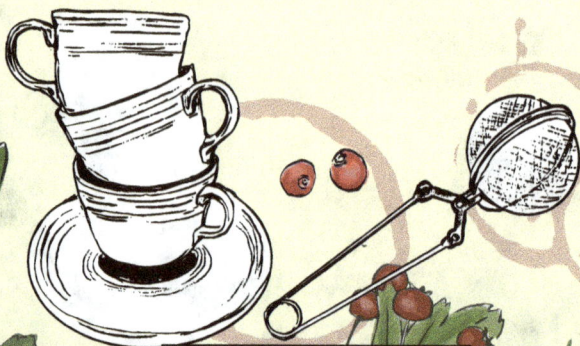

KID FRIENDLY

Rooty Schisandra
TEA BLEND

If you're looking for a tea that packs an undeniable flavor punch, this one is it! Filled with tasty adaptogenic botanicals, this blend of roots and berries will help strengthen the body's systems so it can better withstand stress and change that comes your way in everyday life.

Yield: Approximately four 8 fl oz servings

INGREDIENTS

1 tbsp schisandra (*Schisandra chinensis*) fruit

1 tbsp licorice (*Glycyrrhiza glabra*) root

2 tsp ginger (*Zingiber officinale*) rhizome

2 tsp eleuthero (*Eleutherococcus senticosus*) root

1 tsp astragalus (*Astragalus mongholicus*) root (optional)

1 tsp elder (*Sambucus nigra* or *S. canadensis*) berry

40 fl oz (1.2 L) water

DIRECTIONS

Place herbs in a saucepan with water.

Bring to a boil, cover, then reduce the heat to a simmer.

Simmer for 20 minutes.

Remove from heat, strain decoction into a heat-safe container using a tea strainer, and compost or discard plant material.

Consume immediately or within 48 hours after straining, if refrigerated.

Drink up to four servings per day.

Vani-Tea

Give yourself a glow up with this tea blend packed with nutrient-rich botanicals that are strengthening and nourishing to the hair, skin, and nails when drunk regularly.

Yield: 1⅝ cups dried tea blend

INGREDIENTS

½ cup alfalfa (*Medicago sativa*) aerial parts

½ cup violet (*Viola odorata* or *V. sororia*) leaf

¼ cup peppermint (*Mentha × piperita*) leaf

¼ cup nettle (*Urtica dioica*) leaf

2 tbsp plantain (*Plantago* spp.) leaf

DIRECTIONS

Combine all ingredients and store the blend in a labeled, tightly sealed storage container. Use within 12 months.

Steep ½ cup of tea blend per 32 fl oz (960 mL) freshly boiled hot water in a heat-safe container, covered, for 1-4 hours or overnight.

Strain infusion through a tea strainer and compost or discard plant material.

Rewarm if desired, or serve over ice and enjoy!

Consume immediately or within 24 hours after straining, if refrigerated.

Drink up to four 8 fl oz servings per day.

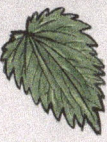

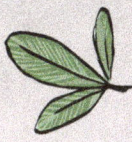

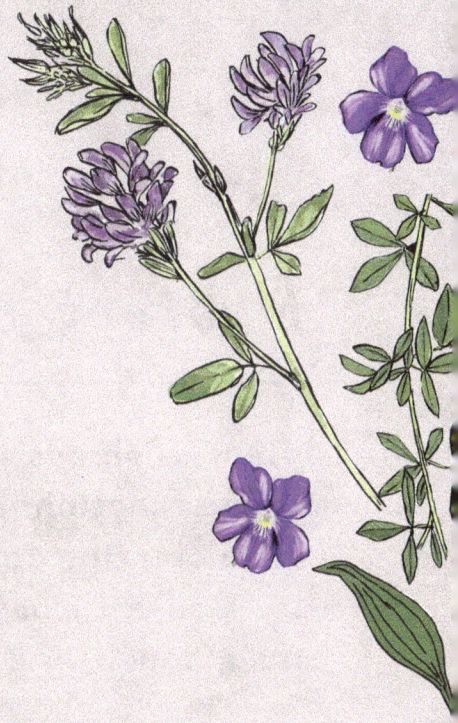

Taking your time to slow down, sip a cup of tea, and be mindful can go a long way in decreasing the stresses of the day.

HERBAL ACADEMY

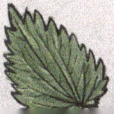

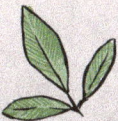

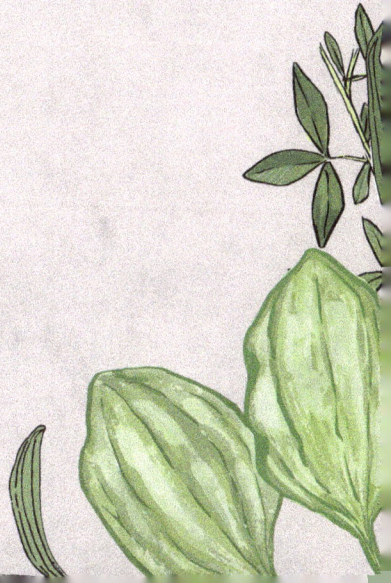

Protect & Soothe

Botanical blends that support healthy immune function, provide a boost when you're starting to feel under the weather, ease a sore throat, get congestion moving, calm a cough, and soothe a fever.

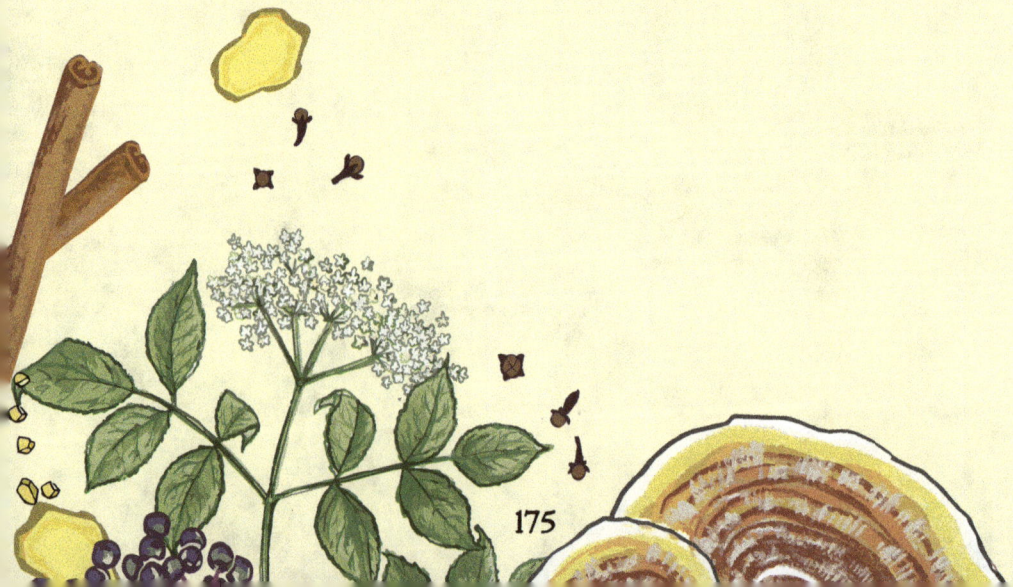

175

RECICES:

Abuelita's
SORE THROAT TEA

When I was growing up, my *abuelita* (grandmother) would prepare honey and lime juice in hot water anytime someone in the family had a hoarse or sore throat. It's a traditional recipe used in Latin America and across the world. Early in my herbal journey, I learned sage is especially useful for a sore or irritated throat, and it seemed like a perfect addition to my abuelita's preparation. Now it's become one of my go-tos for a sore throat, and one day, I'll share it with my *nietos* (grandchildren)!
- Cristina Asensio Foley

Yield: One 8 fl oz serving

INGREDIENTS

3-4 fresh sage (*Salvia officinalis*) leaves

1 tbsp (15 mL) lime juice, freshly squeezed (about ½ of a lime)

1 tbsp (15 mL) honey

8 fl oz (240 mL) water

DIRECTIONS

Place sage and lime juice in a heat-safe container.

Pour freshly boiled hot water over the sage and lime juice, cover, and steep for 5-10 minutes.

Strain the infusion through a tea strainer and compost or discard plant material.

Add honey.

Serve and enjoy!

Drink up to four servings per day.

Boggy Lung Cough
TEA BLEND

This blend is for those struggling with a wet, productive cough that leaves the chest feeling heavy, boggy, and full of thick, stuck mucus. Naturally drying and warming, it encourages expectoration, eases mucous production, and tones the airways.

Yield: Approximately four 8 fl oz servings

INGREDIENTS

8 tsp anise (*Pimpinella anisum*) seed, crushed

4 tsp elecampane (*Inula helenium*) root

4 tsp mullein (*Verbascum thapsus*) leaf

40 fl oz (1.2 L) water

DIRECTIONS

Place all herbs in a saucepan with water.

Bring to a boil, cover, then reduce the heat to a simmer.

Simmer for 20 minutes.

Remove from heat, strain decoction into a heat-safe container using a tea strainer lined with an unbleached coffee filter to ensure the removal of tiny mullein leaf hairs, which can cause irritation, and compost or discard plant material.

Consume immediately or within 48 hours after straining, if refrigerated.

Drink up to four servings per day.

Cacao ImmuniTea

Support healthy immune function in a tasty way with cacao, elderberry, and other immunomodulating herbs. It's the berry botanical hot cocoa you didn't know you needed!

Yield: Approximately two 8 fl oz servings

INGREDIENTS

3 tbsp roasted cacao (*Theobroma cacao*) powder or nibs

2 tbsp astragalus (*Astragalus mongholicus*) root

I tbsp elder (*Sambucus nigra* or *S. canadensis*) berry (or I tsp (5 mL) elderberry syrup)

I stick cinnamon (*Cinnamomum* spp.) bark, crushed

24 fl oz (720 mL) water

Milk of choice (dairy or non-dairy) to taste (optional)

Honey (or sweetener of choice) to taste (optional)

I tsp reishi (*Ganoderma* spp.), cordyceps (*Cordyceps militaris* or *Ophiocordyceps sinensis*), or other immune-boosting mushroom extract powder (optional)

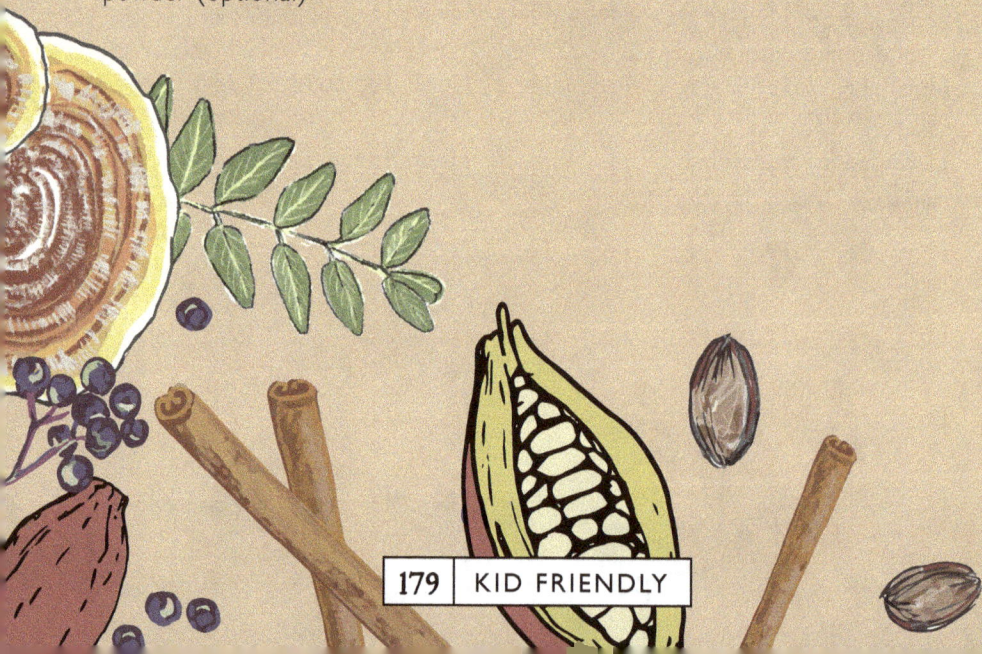

DIRECTIONS

Place all herbs, except elderberry syrup and mushrooms, if using, in a saucepan with water.

Bring to a boil, cover, then reduce the heat to a simmer.

Simmer for 20 minutes.

Remove from heat, strain decoction into a heat-safe container using a tea strainer, and compost or discard plant material.

Add milk, honey, elderberry syrup, and mushroom extract powder, if desired, and stir well to combine.

Serve and enjoy!

Drink up to four servings per day.

CINNAMON
ELDERBERRY TEA

If you're looking for an easy, fruity spiced tea, then we have you covered with this immune-supportive blend. You can enjoy this tea anytime, but it's especially helpful if you have recently been exposed to unwanted germs or eaten a big, heavy meal.

Yield: Two 8 fl oz servings

INGREDIENTS

1 tbsp elder (*Sambucus nigra* or *S. canadensis*) berry

1 tsp tulsi (*Ocimum tenuiflorum*) aerial parts

1 tsp orange (*Citrus* spp.) peel

½ stick cinnamon (*Cinnamomum* spp.) bark, crushed

16 fl oz (480 mL) water

DIRECTIONS

Place herbs in a heat-safe container.

Pour freshly boiled hot water over the herbs, cover, and steep for 15-20 minutes.

Strain the infusion through a tea strainer and compost or discard plant material.

Serve and enjoy!

Drink up to four servings per day.

Jill's Favorite
SICK DAY TEA

The days of suffering for weeks from colds ended when I started drinking this tea at the first sign of symptoms. Full of antibacterial and antiviral components, and high in vitamin C, this tea supports both lung and immune health. As an immunostimulant, echinacea is best employed for acute use.
- Jill York

Yield: 2 cups dried tea blend

INGREDIENTS

½ cup echinacea (*Echinacea* spp.) root

½ cup mullein (*Verbascum thapsus*) leaf

¼ cup peppermint (*Mentha* x *piperita*) leaf

¼ cup rose (*Rosa* spp.) hip

¼ cup elder (*Sambucus nigra* or *S. canadensis*) berry

¼ cup chickweed (*Stellaria media*) aboveground parts

DIRECTIONS

Combine all ingredients and store the blend in a labeled, tightly sealed storage container. Use within 12 months.

Steep 1 tbsp of tea blend per 8 fl oz (240 mL) freshly boiled hot water in a heat-safe container, covered, for 15-20 minutes.

Strain the infusion through a tea strainer lined with an unbleached coffee filter to ensure the removal of tiny mullein leaf hairs, which can cause irritation, and compost or discard plant material.

Drink up to four 8 fl oz servings per day.

Cough-B-Gone Tea

Mullein has long been used to soothe coughs and other respiratory issues because of its anti-inflammatory, antispasmodic, and expectorant properties. The addition of antispasmodic chamomile, demulcent marshmallow, and honey makes this tea very helpful for soothing irritated throats and dry coughs.

Yield: One 12 fl oz serving

INGREDIENTS

1 tbsp chamomile (*Matricaria chamomilla*) flower

1 tsp marshmallow (*Althaea officinalis*) root, leaf, or flower

1 tsp plantain (*Plantago* spp.) leaf

1 tsp mullein (*Verbascum thapsus*) leaf

1 tsp licorice (*Glycyrrhiza glabra*) root

12 fl oz (360 mL) water

Honey (or sweetener of choice) to taste

DIRECTIONS

Place herbs in a heat-safe container.

Pour freshly boiled hot water over the herbs, cover, and steep for 5-7 minutes.

Strain the infusion through a tea strainer lined with an unbleached coffee filter to ensure the removal of tiny mullein leaf hairs, which can cause irritation, and compost or discard plant material.

Sweeten with honey, if desired.

Serve and enjoy!

Drink up to three servings per day.

Elderberry-Ginger Syrup Tea

Wait! What? Elderberry syrup tea? Why, yes ... you read that right! Sip on your favorite traditional immune support preparation (without the added sugar) at the first sign of viral infection. Fresh ginger is one of herbalism's most potent antiviral allies, and alongside elder's immune-stimulating berries, this blend is crafted to support the immune system in its fight against any virus one might be up against. As an immunostimulant, echinacea is best employed for acute use.

Yield: Approximately six 4 fl oz servings

INGREDIENTS

¼ cup elder (*Sambucus nigra* or *S. canadensis*) berry

2-inch piece fresh ginger (*Zingiber officinale*) rhizome, grated

2 tbsp echinacea (*Echinacea* spp.) root

1 tsp cinnamon (*Cinnamomum* spp.) bark, crushed

3 whole clove (*Syzygium aromaticum*) buds

32 fl oz (960 mL) water

Honey (or sweetener of choice) (optional)

DIRECTIONS

Place all herbs in a saucepan with water.

Bring to a boil, cover, then reduce the heat to a simmer.

Simmer for 20 minutes.

Remove from heat, strain decoction into a heat-safe container using a tea strainer, and compost or discard plant material.

Sweeten with honey, if desired.

Consume immediately or within 48 hours after straining, if refrigerated.

Drink up to six servings per day, one 4 fl oz serving every 2-3 hours.

FEVER-COOLING TEA

When a fever is uncomfortably high, herbs can help the body cool down in a gentle, natural way. This fever-cooling tea recipe is filled with antimicrobial herbs that also stimulate the circulatory system and encourage the body to sweat by moving heat from the center of the body outward. If you don't have hyssop or eucalyptus, feel free to sub in yarrow aerial parts or peppermint leaf.

Yield: Eight 2 fl oz servings

INGREDIENTS

2 tsp elder (*Sambucus nigra* or *S. canadensis*) flower

2 tsp eucalyptus (*Eucalyptus globulus*) leaf

1 tsp feverfew (*Tanacetum parthenium*) aerial parts

1 tsp hyssop (*Hyssopus officinalis*) aerial parts

16 fl oz (480 mL) water

Honey (or sweetener of choice) (optional)

DIRECTIONS

Place herbs in a heat-safe container.

Pour freshly boiled hot water over the herbs, cover, and steep for 15-20 minutes.

Strain the infusion through a tea strainer and compost or discard plant material.

Sweeten with honey, if desired.

Serve hot and enjoy!

Drink up to eight servings per day, one 2 fl oz serving every 30 minutes.

FOREST TEA

My maternal grandmother dwelled on these hills I call home long before me and, taking notice of what grew around her, every winter she brewed her family cups of pine needle tea to help ward off colds and respiratory infections. Even though she couldn't read or write, firsthand experience and passed-down knowledge told her she was doing something right. In fact, pine needles are high in vitamin C and count expectorant and decongestant properties among their actions. This tea recipe is deeply inspired by her, with a couple of herbal additions for a warming and aromatic blend.
- Catarina Seixas

Yield: Three 8 fl oz servings

INGREDIENTS

2 tbsp fresh pine (*Pinus* spp.) needle, gently crushed

1 tbsp fresh orange peel, chopped

1 stick cinnamon (*Cinnamomum* spp.) bark, crushed

24 fl oz (720 mL) water

Honey (or sweetener of choice) to taste (optional)

DIRECTIONS

Place herbs in a heat-safe container.

Pour freshly boiled hot water over the herbs, cover, and steep for 15-20 minutes.

Strain the infusion through a tea strainer and compost or discard plant material.

Sweeten with honey, if desired.

Consume immediately or within 24 hours after straining, if refrigerated.

Drink up to three servings per day.

KID FRIENDLY

Ginger
FLOWER POWER TEA

Fresh ginger juice is a go-to for any viral infection due to its strong antiviral action. Pair that with the relaxing effects of elder flower, and you've got yourself a powerful duo when the next viral ailment comes your way. This makes a potent drink to be taken in small amounts several times per day; feel free to dilute each serving with a few fluid ounces of hot water if preferred OR feel free to double the amount of ginger if you want to amp up the potency!

Yield: Approximately five 2 fl oz servings

INGREDIENTS

2-inch long piece fresh ginger (*Zingiber officinale*) rhizome

1 tbsp elder (*Sambucus nigra* or *S. canadensis*) flower

1 tbsp (15 mL) lemon juice, freshly squeezed

10-12 fl oz (300-360 mL) water

1-3 tsp (5-15 mL) honey (or sweetener of choice)

DIRECTIONS

Method 1:

Using a juicer, process the ginger and capture the juice (a 2-inch long piece produces approximately 2 tbsp fresh ginger juice). Set aside. If you don't have a juicer, see directions in Method 2.

Pour 10 fl oz (300 mL) freshly boiled hot water over the elder flower, cover, and steep for 10 minutes.

Remove from heat, strain infusion into a heat-safe container using a tea strainer, and compost or discard plant material.

Add 2 tbsp of the reserved ginger juice, along with the lemon juice and honey, and stir well to combine.

Store any remaining ginger juice in the refrigerator for your next serving within 24 hours, or freeze in an ice cube tray for later use.

Drink five servings per day, one 2 fl oz serving every 2-3 hours.

KID FRIENDLY

Method 2:

Grate ginger.

Place 12 fl oz (360 mL) water in a saucepan. Add grated ginger and bring to a boil, cover, then reduce the heat to a simmer.

Simmer for 10 minutes.

Turn off heat, add elder flower, and let steep for 10 minutes.

Remove from heat, strain decoction into a heat-safe container using a tea strainer, and compost or discard plant material.

Add lemon juice and honey, and stir well to combine.

Drink five servings per day, one serving every 2-3 hours.

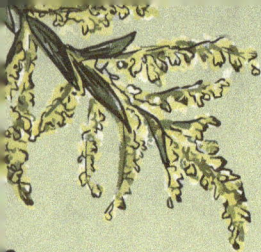

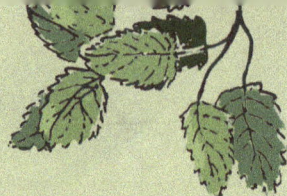

golden green tea

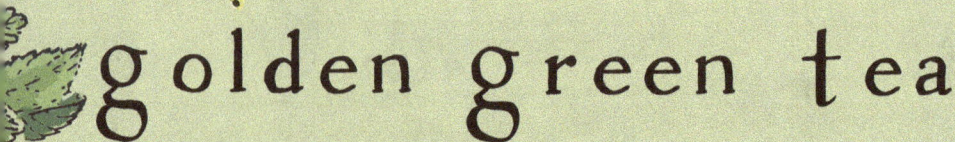

Goldenrod is ubiquitous, overlooked, and unfairly maligned as a cause of seasonal allergies (it's not), all at the same time! Herbalists harness its astringent, antimicrobial, and diaphoretic qualities to tone and dry tissues, ease seasonal allergies and respiratory infections, and help sweat out fever. This blend offers a slightly bitter, astringent, and sweet taste from goldenrod, and the overall flavor profile is brightened up with the addition of mint leaves. Try this simple tea and you may be surprised at the support it has to offer!

Yield: Two 8 fl oz servings

INGREDIENTS

1 tbsp goldenrod (*Solidago* spp.) aerial parts

1 tbsp mint (*Mentha* spp.) leaf

16 fl oz (480 mL) water

DIRECTIONS

Place herbs in a heat-safe container.

Pour freshly boiled hot water over the herbs, cover, and steep for 15 minutes.

Strain the infusion through a tea strainer and compost or discard plant material.

Serve and enjoy!

Drink up to four servings per day.

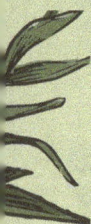

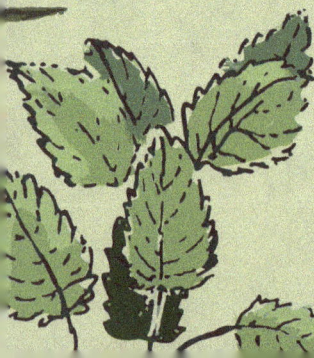

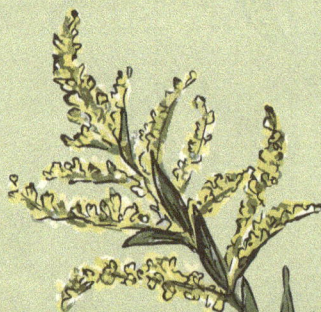

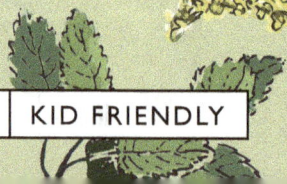

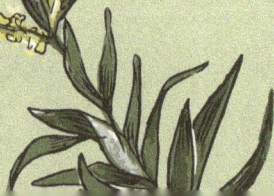

| KID FRIENDLY

HIGH-C IMMUNE BOOSTING TEA

Whenever seasonal bugs are spreading, giving the immune system a boost is key to support the body's defenses against viral illnesses. Herbs rich in vitamin C can be part of your herbal protocol for supporting the immune system and keeping viruses at bay! Pour yourself a mug of this tea often to sip all through cold and flu season.

Yield: 1⅝ cups dried tea blend

INGREDIENTS

½ cup hibiscus (*Hibiscus sabdariffa*) calyx

½ cup rose (*Rosa* spp.) hip

¼ cup lemongrass (*Cymbopogon citratus*) leaf

¼ cup lemon (*Citrus* x *limon*) peel

2 tbsp cinnamon (*Cinnamomum* spp.) bark, crushed

DIRECTIONS

Combine all ingredients and store the blend in a labeled, tightly sealed storage container. Use within 12 months.

Steep 1 tbsp of tea blend per 8 fl oz (240 mL) freshly boiled hot water in a heat-safe container, covered, for 10-15 minutes.

Strain infusion through a tea strainer and compost or discard plant material.

Serve and enjoy!

Drink up to three 8 fl oz servings per day.

RESPIRATORY
reinforcement tea

This gentle tea blend can be just the thing to help soothe and assist the body when dealing with a respiratory virus. The herbs in this blend act as a gentle expectorant, assisting the body in expelling excess or stuck respiratory mucus, soothe a sore throat, and gently encourage resolution of fever. The licorice adds a slightly sweet flavor that can be appealing to reticent tea drinkers; for those who don't love the taste of licorice, marshmallow root can be used as a substitute.

Yield: 1½ cups dried tea blend

INGREDIENTS

¾ cup tulsi (*Ocimum tenuiflorum*) aerial parts

¼ cup + 2 tbsp mullein (*Verbascum thapsus*) leaf

3 tbsp licorice (*Glycyrrhiza glabra*) root

3 tbsp elder (*Sambucus nigra* or *S. canadensis*) flower

DIRECTIONS

Combine all ingredients and store the blend in a labeled, tightly sealed storage container. Use within 12 months.

Steep 1 tbsp of tea blend per 8 fl oz (240 mL) freshly boiled hot water in a heat-safe container, covered, for 15-20 minutes.

Strain the infusion through a tea strainer lined with an unbleached coffee filter to ensure the removal of tiny mullein leaf hairs, which can cause irritation, and compost or discard plant material.

Serve and enjoy!

Drink up to four 8 fl oz servings per day.

Stacy's
Black Currant Boost

Growing up in Australia, warm black currant tea was served whenever we felt the sniffles coming on. This comforting blend of tart flavors incorporates black currants, rose hips, and hibiscus, which are high in antioxidants and vitamin C to bolster your immune system.
- Stacy Karen

Yield: Approximately four 8 fl oz servings

INGREDIENTS

1 cup dried black currant fruit

1 tbsp hibiscus (*Hibiscus sabdariffa*) calyx

1 tbsp rose (*Rosa* spp.) hip

Honey (or sweetener of choice) to taste (optional)

40 fl oz (1200 mL) water

DIRECTIONS

Place black currant and hibiscus in a saucepan with water.

Bring to a boil, cover, then reduce the heat to a simmer.

Simmer for 20 minutes.

Remove from heat, add rose hips, cover, and steep for another 10 minutes.

Strain decoction into a heat-safe container using a tea strainer, and compost or discard plant material.

Add honey to taste, if desired.

Sip hot, or allow to cool and serve over ice.

Consume immediately or within 48 hours after straining, if refrigerated.

Drink up to four servings per day.

CHAPTER FIVE
TEA LATTES, MATCHA, AND CHAI BLENDS

Herbs lend themselves well to favorite specialty drinks such as lattes, chai, and matcha blends that are popular in coffee shops for good reason—depending on whether they are hot or cold, they can be cozy or refreshing, but they are always satisfying! You can take these preparations to the next level by adding adaptogens, calming nervines, and glorious herbal flourishes (lavender cold foam, anyone?), and they produce ooh-la-la-licious results!

We've flipped one latte recipe on its head with calming herbs—not a speck of caffeine to be found in our Cham-a-Calming Latte so it can be enjoyed day or night—and we've rounded out matcha teas with rose, lavender, or adaptogens—just take your pick! Our love letter to chai includes not one, not two, but four favorite versions of this spicy, warming, herb-forward traditional drink. And we finish with a final ode to the moon with a rose (*Rosa* spp.), cardamom (*Elettaria cardamomum*), and fennel (*Foeniculum vulgare*) blend that brings lusciousness and uplift during the dark of the new moon.

CHAM-*a*-CALMING LATTE

Support a healthy stress response with this latte tea recipe filled with adaptogen and relaxing nervine botanicals to strengthen, tone, and nourish the body so it can better handle changes that come its way.

Yield: One 8 fl oz serving

INGREDIENTS

4 fl oz (120 mL) water

1 tbsp rose (*Rosa* spp.) petal

1 tbsp chamomile (*Matricaria chamomilla*) flower

1 tsp ginger (*Zingiber officinale*) rhizome

¼ tsp reishi (*Ganoderma* spp.) mushroom extract, powdered

¼ tsp ashwagandha (*Withania somnifera*) root, powdered

4 fl oz (120 mL) milk of choice (dairy or non-dairy)

½ tsp (2.5 mL) vanilla extract

1 tsp (5 mL) honey (or sweetener of choice)

DIRECTIONS

Place chamomile, rose, and ginger in a heat-safe container.

Pour freshly boiled hot water over the herbs, cover, and steep for 3-5 minutes.

Strain the infusion through a tea strainer and compost or discard plant material.

Transfer liquid to a high-speed blender, add remaining ingredients, and blend until smooth and frothy.

Serve and enjoy!

Drink up to four servings per day.

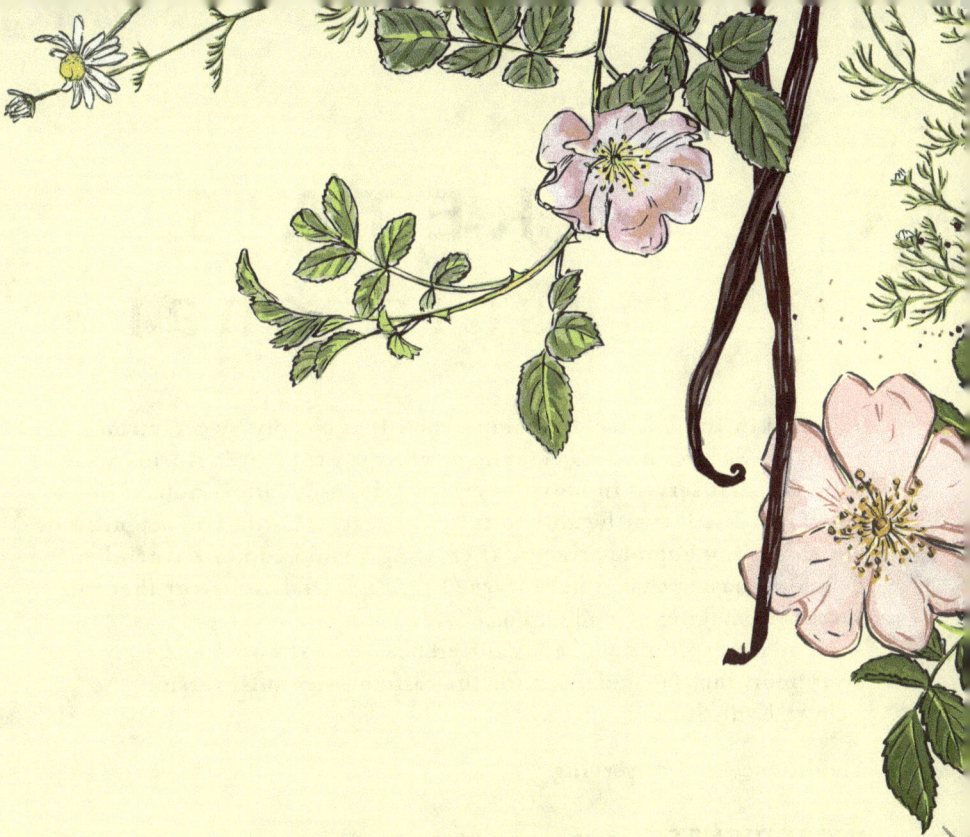

Willowy, fragrant, soothing
chamomile – you had me
at hello!

MARLENE ADELMANN

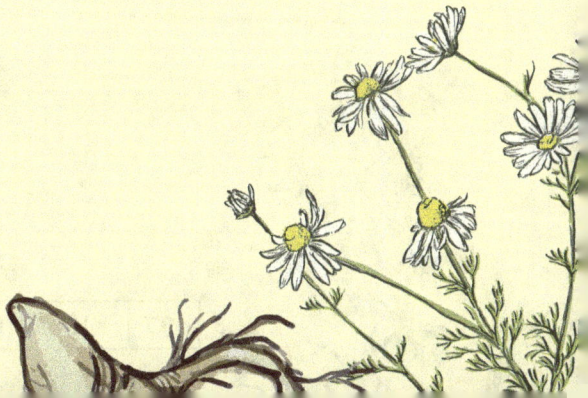

GRETA'S
masala chai

The chai in India is truly incomparable. It is creamy, sweet, strong, and aromatic. Served in small ceramic or glass tea cups, it is worlds away from the chai served in most American cafes and coffee shops. I don't know that I will ever be able to fully replicate its aromatic magnificence, but this is my humble attempt at creating a good cup of flavorful and delicious masala chai. I have learned through trial and error that the success in making a good cup of chai lies largely in the process. Also, good quality spices make a big difference. This is how I make my chai every morning. For kids, opt for the caffeine-free tulsi version.
- Greta Kent-Stoll

Yield: One 12 fl oz serving

INGREDIENTS

6 fl oz (180 mL) water

6 fl oz (180 mL) milk of choice (dairy or non-dairy)

1 tbsp CTC (cut, torn, curled) black Assam tea (or tulsi (*Ocimum tenuiflorum*) aerial parts for a caffeine-free option)

½ tsp ginger (*Zingiber officinale*) rhizome, powdered

¼ tsp cinnamon (*Cinnamomum* spp.) bark, powdered

¼ tsp cardamom (*Elettaria cardamomum*) seed, powdered

1 large pinch black pepper (*Piper nigrum*) fruit, powdered

1 pinch clove (*Syzygium aromaticum*) bud, powdered

Honey (or sweetener of choice) to taste

DIRECTIONS

Place water, milk, and spices in a saucepan.

Bring just to a slight boil.

Remove from heat, add black tea (or tulsi), cover, and steep for 2-5 minutes.

Strain infusion into a heat-safe container using a tea strainer, and compost or discard plant material.

Sweeten with honey.

Serve with a pinch more of cardamom and enjoy!

Drink up to four servings per day.

NOTES

CTC Assam is sold in most Indian markets, as well as specialty tea shops and online suppliers. However, if you have a hard time tracking some down, you can substitute whole leaf Assam, Darjeeling, or English breakfast tea. In this case, use 2 tablespoons of loose leaf tea.

Using powdered spices is easy and convenient. However, you can add a bit of freshly grated ginger rhizome to this recipe, as well as a few crushed cardamom pods. Add these whole spices at the same time as the powdered spices.

heart opening
MATCHA

I will often switch out my morning cuppa coffee with matcha in the early spring or lean on it for an afternoon pick me up. I love infusing the water used to make matcha with herbal goodness. I tend to lean on damiana for its stimulating effects and it really gives me support with grounding in my body and connecting socially and emotionally with others. Along with the heart tending power of rose, they work together in this blend to create an inviting, uplifting, opening effect. For a caffeine-free option, replace the matcha with powdered nettle leaf.
- Alyson Morgan

Yield: Approximately three 8 fl oz servings

INGREDIENTS

1 tsp damiana (*Turnera diffusa*) aerial parts

1 tsp rose (*Rosa* spp.) petal

1 cardamom (*Elettaria cardamomum*) pod, crushed

16 fl oz (480 mL) water

4-8 tsp matcha (*Camellia sinensis*) leaf powder (or nettle (*Urtica dioica*) leaf, powdered, for a caffeine-free option)

16 fl oz (480 mL) milk of choice (dairy or non-dairy)

Honey (or sweetener of choice) to taste (optional)

DIRECTIONS

Place herbs except matcha in a saucepan with 16 fl oz (480 mL) water and 16 fl oz (480 mL) milk of choice (dairy or non-dairy).

Bring to a boil, cover, then reduce the heat to a simmer.

Simmer for 10 minutes.

Remove from heat, strain decoction into a heat-safe container using a tea strainer, and compost or discard herbal material.

Sift matcha into a small bowl, cover with decoction and whisk until frothy.

Add honey, if desired.

Serve and enjoy!

Consume immediately or within 48 hours after straining, if refrigerated.

Drink up three 8 fl oz servings per day.

HERBAL CHAI FOR ALL

A mug of this herbal chai is a warm and welcoming beverage to help you return to a centered place, and find a home within yourself.

Yield: Approximately six 8 fl oz servings

INGREDIENTS

48 fl oz (1.4 L) water

14 cardamom (*Elettaria cardamomum*) pods, crushed

12 clove (*Syzygium aromaticum*) buds, crushed

16 black pepper (*Piper nigrum*) fruits, crushed

2-3 sticks cinnamon (*Cinnamomum* spp.) bark, crushed

4 fresh ginger (*Zingiber officinale*) rhizome slices

½ tbsp astragalus (*Astragalus mongholicus*) root, powdered

½ tbsp rose (*Rosa* spp.) hip

½ tbsp tulsi (*Ocimum tenuiflorum*) aerial parts

½-1 tsp fennel (*Foeniculum vulgare*) seed

8-16 fl oz (240-480 mL) milk of choice (dairy or non-dairy)

Honey (or sweetener of choice) to taste

DIRECTIONS

Place all herbs, except rose hip, tulsi, and fennel, in a saucepan with water.

Bring to a boil, cover, then reduce the heat to a simmer.

Simmer for 20 minutes.

Remove from heat, add rose hip, tulsi, and fennel, cover, and steep for another 5 minutes.

Strain decoction into a heat-safe container using a tea strainer, and compost or discard plant material.

Add milk and honey.

Serve and enjoy!

Consume immediately or within 48 hours after straining, if refrigerated.

Drink up to four servings per day.

IMMUNE
boosting chai

Warm up with a tasty drink that feels more like a treat than something healthy for you. This botanical brew features roots, spices, pods, and peels that all support the immune system so it can keep you healthy and happy when cold and flu season rolls around. For kids, opt for the caffeine-free raspberry leaf version.

Yield: Approximately two 8 fl oz servings

INGREDIENTS

16 fl oz (480 mL) water

2 tsp astragalus (*Astragalus mongholicus*) root

6 black pepper (*Piper nigrum*) fruits, crushed

4 cardamom (*Elettaria cardamomum*) pods, crushed

3 clove (*Syzygium aromaticum*) buds, crushed

1 slice ginger (*Zingiber officinale*) rhizome, fresh

2 sticks cinnamon (*Cinnamomum* spp.) bark, crushed

1 tsp orange (*Citrus* spp.) peel

4-8 fl oz (120-240 mL) milk of choice (dairy or non-dairy)

1 tbsp loose black tea (*Camellia sinensis*) leaf (or two tea bags) (or raspberry (*Rubus idaeus*) leaf for a caffeine-free option)

Honey (or sweetener of choice) to taste (optional)

DIRECTIONS

Place astragalus in a saucepan with 16 fl oz (480 mL) water.

Bring to a boil, cover, then reduce the heat to a simmer.

Simmer for 20 minutes.

Add spices and milk, cover, and simmer for another 5 minutes.

Remove from heat, add tea (or raspberry), and steep for 10 minutes.

Strain decoction into a heat-safe container using a tea strainer, and compost or discard plant material.

Add honey, if desired.

Serve and enjoy!

Drink up to four servings per day.

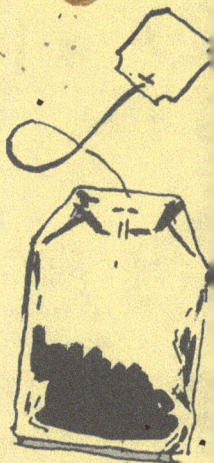

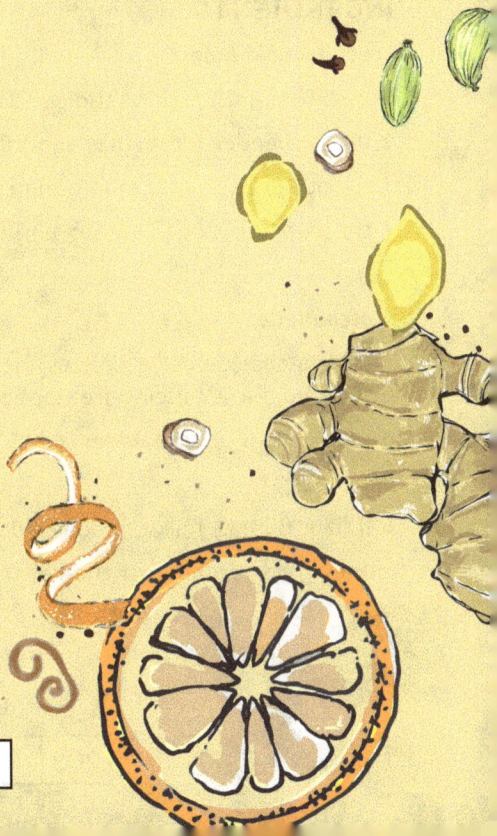

ICED *lavender*
MATCHA LATTE

With a long history of use in traditional Japanese tea ceremonies, matcha is a type of green tea with many wonderful benefits. Matcha tea is made by grinding the shade-grown *Camellia sinensis* leaves into a fine powder, which differs from the green tea many of us enjoy, prepared by steeping the leaves in hot water. Matcha allows us to consume the leaves themselves, in powdered form, rather than as an infusion. Along with antioxidant and anti-inflammatory properties, matcha has long been regarded for its ability to help with clarity of mind and focus and guard against neurodegenerative disorders. Fast forward to this recipe ... with less sugar than its popular commercial version and no additives, we love this homemade twist on this refreshing drink! For kids, opt for the caffeine-free nettle version.

Yield: Two 9 fl oz servings

INGREDIENTS
Lavender cold foam:

8 fl oz (240 mL) milk of choice (dairy or non-dairy)

½ tbsp lavender (*Lavandula* spp.) flower bud

I tsp butterfly pea (*Clitoria ternatea*) flower

I tsp black currant (*Ribes nigrum*) fruit, powdered

Matcha latte:

I tsp matcha (*Camellia sinensis*) powder (or nettle (*Urtica dioica*) leaf, powdered, for a caffeine-free option)

4 fl oz (120 mL) cold water

Ice cubes

6 fl oz (180 mL) milk of choice (dairy or non-dairy)

Honey (or sweetener of choice) to taste

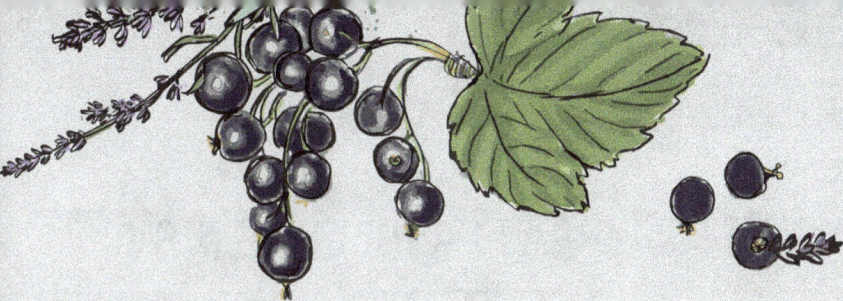

DIRECTIONS

Place lavender cold foam ingredients in a glass jar, stir well, cap, and steep overnight in the refrigerator.

Strain infused milk using a tea strainer, and compost or discard plant material.

Use a milk frother to froth infused milk and set aside.

Sift matcha into a small bowl, cover with cold water, and whisk until frothy.

Add ice cubes to a glass jar.

Pour cold milk over ice followed by frothed matcha.

Sweeten with honey, and stir well to combine.

Top with frothed lavender cold foam, serve, and enjoy!

Drink up to four servings per day.

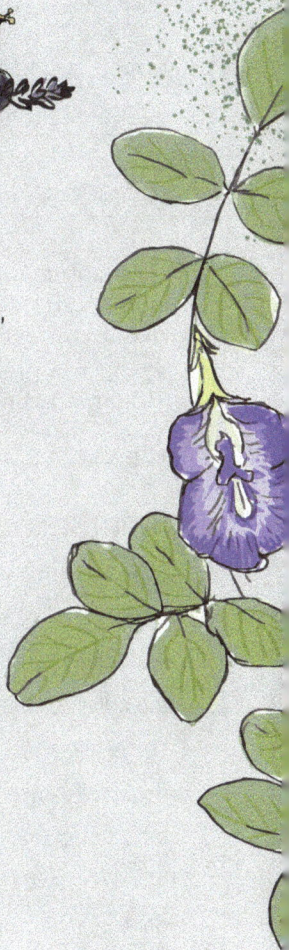

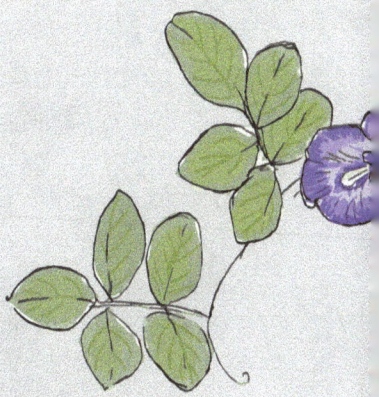

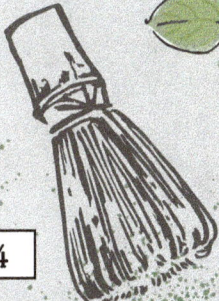

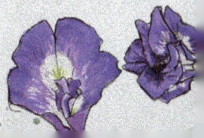

MATCHA & ADAPTOGENS
LATTE

This adaptogenic latte combines the best of both worlds. Matcha contains caffeine and is mildly stimulating. Ashwagandha root is an ayurvedic *rasayana* (deeply rejuvenating herb) and is also considered an adaptogen, as is tulsi. This herbal blend offers gentle stimulation along with botanical nourishment and flavor.

Yield: One 10 fl oz serving

INGREDIENTS

2 fl oz (60 mL) water

1 tsp matcha (*Camellia sinensis*) leaf powder

1 tsp ashwagandha (*Withania somnifera*) root, powdered

1 tsp tulsi (*Ocimum tenuiflorum*) aerial parts, powdered

1 tsp astragalus (*Astragalus mongholicus*) root, powdered

8 fl oz (240 mL) milk of choice (dairy or non-dairy)

1 pinch cinnamon (*Cinnamomum* spp.) bark, powdered

Honey (or sweetener of choice) to taste

1 pinch cardamom (*Elettaria cardamomum*) seed, powdered, for garnish (optional)

DIRECTIONS

Place all finely powdered herbs except cinnamon and cardamom in a heat-safe container.

Pour freshly boiled hot water over the herbs, and whisk until smooth.

Place milk in a saucepan and heat until steaming.

Add milk, honey, and a pinch of cinnamon to the powdered herb mixture, and whisk until smooth.

Serve with a pinch of cardamom powder and enjoy!

Drink up to four servings per day.

NEW MOON
TEA

Prepare this on the morning of a New Moon to give yourself a little bit of upliftment during times of lowered energy. If you enjoy this blend, you don't have to wait until the next New Moon to brew a cup! For kids, opt for the caffeine-free raspberry leaf version.

Yield: Two 8 fl oz servings

INGREDIENTS

8 fl oz (240 mL) water

8 fl oz (240 mL) milk of choice (dairy or non-dairy)

1 tbsp black tea (*Camellia sinensis*) leaf (or 2-3 black tea bags) (or raspberry (*Rubus idaeus*) leaf for a caffeine-free option)

2 tsp rose (*Rosa* spp.) petal

1 tsp fennel (*Foeniculum vulgare*) seed

1 cardamom (*Elettaria cardamomum*) pod, crushed

Honey (or sweetener of choice) to taste

Crushed rose petals, for garnish (optional)

DIRECTIONS

Bring water and milk to a simmer in a saucepan, add black tea, cover, and steep for 2 minutes.

Remove from heat, add herbs, and steep for another 2 minutes.

Strain infusion into a heat-safe container using a tea strainer, and compost or discard plant material.

Add honey.

Serve with a few crushed rose petals, if desired, and enjoy!

Drink up to four servings per day.

Sweet and Spicy Adaptogenic Chai

Looking for a dessert tea to stimulate your palate while strengthening your body? If so, this sweet and spicy adaptogenic chai makes a great morning or evening drink that will do just that very thing. Formulated with circulation-stimulating herbs that pack a punch in the flavor department alongside sweet and balancing adaptogens that benefit the whole body, this recipe is one you'll find yourself coming back to again and again!

Yield: 1¾ cups dried tea blend

INGREDIENTS

½ cup astragalus (*Astragalus mongholicus*) root

½ cup cinnamon (*Cinnamomum* spp.) bark, crushed

¼ cup ginger (*Zingiber officinale*) rhizome

¼ cup orange (*Citrus* spp.) peel

2 tbsp licorice (*Glycyrrhiza glabra*) root

2 tbsp clove (*Syzygium aromaticum*) bud

6-10 cardamom (*Elettaria cardamomum*) pods, crushed

DIRECTIONS

Combine all ingredients and store the blend in a labeled, tightly sealed storage container. Use within 12 months.

Place 2-3 tbsp of chai blend in a saucepan with 8 fl oz (240 mL) water and 8 fl oz (240 mL) milk of choice (dairy or non-dairy).

Bring to a boil, cover, then reduce the heat to a simmer.

Simmer for 10-15 minutes.

Remove from heat, strain decoction into a heat-safe container using a tea strainer, and compost or discard plant material.

Add honey, if desired.

Serve and enjoy!

Drink up three 8 fl oz servings per day.

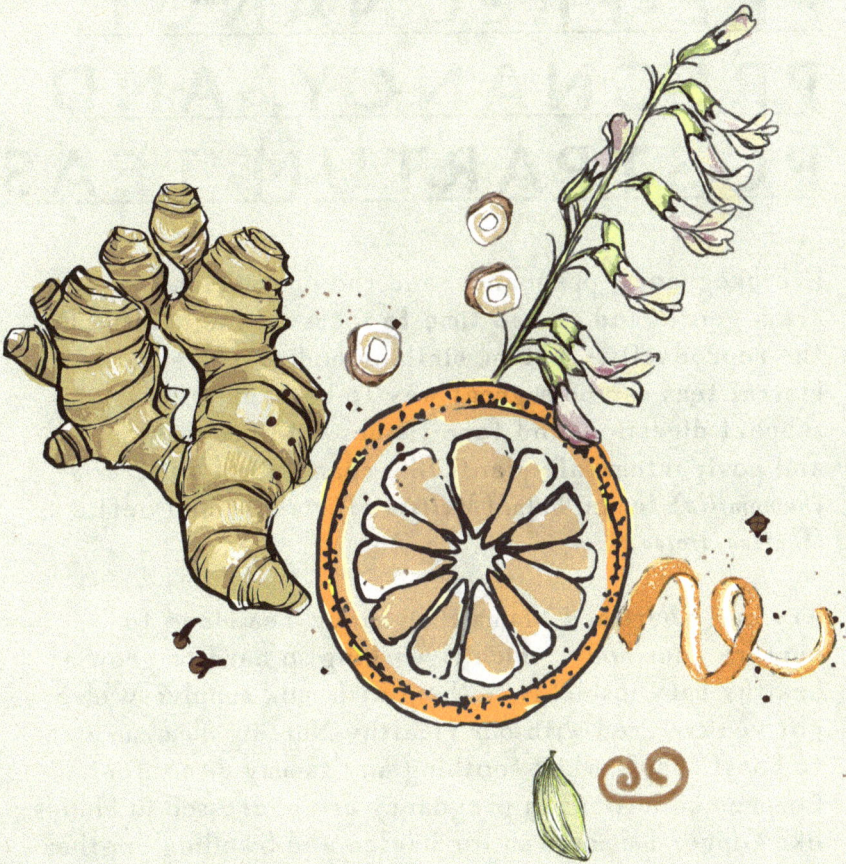

CHAPTER SIX
<u>PRE-PREGNANCY, PREGNANCY, AND POSTPARTUM TEAS</u>

Pre-pregnancy, pregnancy, and the postpartum period are a gentle and sacred time to focus on the health of the reproductive system, birthing bodies, and babies. Herbal teas can be a great way to boost nutrition, support digestion, and tone tissues with pregnancy and postpartum-safe plants like chamomile (*Matricaria chamomilla*), lemon balm (*Melissa officinalis*), and nettle (*Urtica dioica*).

Try our Nourished Mama Pregnancy Tea blend to nurture your body, which is working so hard to grow a healthy baby inside! Need help with milk supply? We've got you covered with our Healthy Nursing Tea, sure to boost supply while soothing any tummy discomfort. Common conditions in pregnancy are addressed in blends like Ginger Lemon Tea for nausea and Swelling Soother Pregnancy Tea to ease fluid retention. These recipes use herbs that are generally considered safe during pregnancy and nursing, though if you choose to use these blends, it is always best practice to do so under the supervision of an experienced midwife, obstetrician herbalist, or medical provider.

cool the burn
TEA

Heartburn is a common symptom during pregnancy, but thankfully these cooling botanicals can help support digestion, cool excess heat, and soothe irritation in the tissues when used regularly in the second and third trimesters.

Yield: Four 8 fl oz servings

INGREDIENTS

1 tbsp spearmint (*Mentha spicata*) leaf

1 tbsp plantain (*Plantago* spp.) leaf

1 tbsp lemon balm (*Melissa officinalis*) aerial parts

2 tsp raspberry (*Rubus* spp.) leaf

1 tsp chamomile (*Matricaria chamomilla*) flower

32 fl oz (960 mL) water

DIRECTIONS

Place herbs in a heat-safe container.

Pour room temperature water over the herbs, cover, and steep for 4 hours to overnight.

Strain the infusion through a tea strainer and compost or discard plant material.

Serve over ice and enjoy!

Drink up to four servings per day.

KID + PREGNANCY FRIENDLY

Good Morning
LIVER DECOCTION

Did you know that supporting liver function and elimination also helps to optimize fertility? This morning liver tea blend is a great place to start if you are thinking about a future pregnancy or trying to conceive.

Yield: Approximately two 8 fl oz servings

INGREDIENTS

2 tsp dandelion (*Taraxacum officinale*) root

2 tsp burdock (*Arctium lappa*) root

1 tsp nettle (*Urtica dioica*) leaf

1 tsp ginger (*Zingiber officinale*) rhizome

32 fl oz (960 mL) water

DIRECTIONS

Place herbs and water in a saucepan.

Bring to a boil, cover, then reduce the heat to a simmer.

Simmer for 20-30 minutes or until the water level reduces to 16 fl oz (480 mL).

Remove from heat, strain decoction into a heat-safe container using a tea strainer, and compost or discard plant material.

Serve and enjoy!

Drink up to two servings per day.

KID FRIENDLY

GINGER
lemon tea

Ginger and lemon are a great way to ease nausea and vomiting during pregnancy. Not only are they safe and effective but they make a tasty pairing for a cup of tea!

Yield: One 8 fl oz serving

INGREDIENTS

1 tsp fresh ginger (*Zingiber officinale*) rhizome, chopped or grated

8 fl oz (240 mL) water

1-2 tsp (5-10 mL) lemon juice, freshly squeezed

DIRECTIONS

Place ginger in a heat-safe container.

Pour freshly boiled hot water over the ginger, cover, and steep for 20 minutes.

Strain the infusion through a tea strainer and compost or discard plant material.

Add freshly squeezed lemon juice to the tea.

Serve and enjoy!

Drink up to two servings per day.

NEW PARENT
HUG IN A MUG

This tea blend is true to its name. It's like getting a hug in a mug as the botanicals in this blend help with stress, energy, and mood support during the postpartum period—and is nice for all the caretakers in the household!

Yield: One 8 fl oz serving

INGREDIENTS

2 tsp linden (*Tilia* spp.) flower and bract

1 tsp chamomile (*Matricaria chamomilla*) flower

1 tsp lemon balm (*Melissa officinalis*) aerial parts

¼ tsp lavender (*Lavandula* spp.) flower bud

8 fl oz (240 mL) water

DIRECTIONS

Place herbs in a heat-safe container.

Pour freshly boiled hot water over the herbs, cover, and steep for 10-20 minutes.

Strain the infusion through a tea strainer and compost or discard plant material.

Serve and enjoy!

Drink up to four servings per day.

healthy *nursing* tea

This delicious herbal blend is a wonderful way to support milk production in the postpartum period. It enables the milk to flow, enriches it with nutrients, and has beneficial properties to soothe baby's tummy discomfort.

Yield: 1¼ cups dried tea blend

INGREDIENTS

¼ cup oat (*Avena sativa*) straw

¼ cup nettle (*Urtica dioica*) leaf

¼ cup alfalfa (*Medicago sativa*) leaf

¼ cup raspberry (*Rubus idaeus*) leaf

2 tbsp fennel (*Foeniculum vulgare*) seed

1 tbsp anise (*Pimpinella anisum*) seed

1 tbsp fenugreek (*Trigonella foenum-graecum*) seed

DIRECTIONS

Combine all ingredients and store the blend in a labeled, tightly sealed storage container. Use within 12 months.

Steep ¼ cup of tea blend per 32 fl oz (960 mL) freshly boiled hot water in a heat-safe container, covered, for 15 minutes.

Strain infusion through a tea strainer and compost or discard plant material.

Serve and enjoy!

Consume immediately or within 24 hours after straining, if refrigerated.

Drink up to four 8 fl oz servings per day.

– nourished mama –
PREGNANCY TEA

This herbal pregnancy tea blend is a wonderful way to boost your intake of iron, calcium, and many vitamins and other trace minerals, keeping you nourished throughout this special time. This pregnancy tea can be enjoyed in the second and third trimester, and also aids as a birth preparation brew.

Yield: 1¼ cups dried tea blend

INGREDIENTS

½ cup raspberry (*Rubus idaeus*) leaf

½ cup nettle (*Urtica dioica*) leaf

¼ cup oat (*Avena sativa*) straw

1 tbsp spearmint (*Mentha spicata*) leaf

DIRECTIONS

Combine all ingredients and store the blend in a labeled, tightly sealed storage container. Use within 12 months.

Steep ¼ cup of tea blend per 32 fl oz (960 mL) freshly boiled hot water in a heat-safe container, covered, for 30 minutes.

Strain infusion through a tea strainer and compost or discard plant material.

Add 2 tbsp lemon juice, freshly squeezed, and sweeten with honey (or sweetener of choice), to taste, if desired.

Sip hot, or allow to cool and serve over ice, and enjoy!

Consume immediately or within 24 hours after straining, if refrigerated.

Drink up to four 8 fl oz servings per day.

NOURISH & TONE
UTERINE TEA

Show the uterus some love with a botanical blend that helps nourish, tone, and tighten the tissues, and can be used pre-pregnancy to prepare this important organ. This tea is also perfect to drink after labor, or the week before menstruation to help ease cramping and pain, and can even be used daily if heavy cramping is common.

Yield: 2 cups dried tea blend

INGREDIENTS

½ cup lady's mantle (*Alchemilla vulgaris*) aerial parts

½ cup raspberry (*Rubus idaeus*) leaf

¼ cup tulsi (*Ocimum tenuiflorum*) aerial parts

¼ cup lemon balm (*Melissa officinalis*) aerial parts

¼ cup plantain (*Plantago* spp.) leaf

¼ cup marshmallow (*Althaea officinalis*) or hollyhock (*Alcea rosea*) leaf

DIRECTIONS

Combine all ingredients and store the blend in a labeled, tightly sealed storage container. Use within 12 months.

Steep 1 tbsp of tea blend per 8 fl oz (240 mL) freshly boiled hot water in a heat-safe container, covered, for 10 minutes.

Strain infusion through a tea strainer and compost or discard plant material.

Sip hot, or allow to cool and serve over ice, and enjoy!

Drink up to four 8 fl oz servings per day.

SWELLING SOOTHER
pregnancy tea

It's not uncommon to experience fluid retention toward the end of pregnancy, leading to swollen hands and feet. After speaking to your doctor to ensure there are no serious underlying causes and sharing the herbs you wish to take, enjoy a couple glasses of this tasty tea to support healthy fluid levels.

Yield: One 8 fl oz serving

INGREDIENTS

1 tsp nettle (*Urtica dioica*) leaf

1 tsp corn (*Zea mays*) pistil (silk)

1 tsp dandelion (*Taraxacum officinale*) leaf

8 fl oz (240 mL) water

DIRECTIONS

Place herbs in a heat-safe container.

Pour freshly boiled hot water over the herbs, cover, and steep for 15-20 minutes.

Strain the infusion through a tea strainer and compost or discard plant material.

Serve and enjoy!

Drink up to two servings per day.

vessel
RESCUE TEA

Pregnancy can put a strain on blood vessels due to extra blood volume common during this time. Thankfully, antioxidant-rich botanicals used in pre-pregnancy can provide some strength and support and help offset the chance of unwelcome blood vessel related conditions occurring during pregnancy. This blend is also supportive post-pregnancy to tone blood vessels. Swap in nettle leaf for a caffeine-free option.

Yield: One 8 fl oz serving

INGREDIENTS

1 tsp green tea (*Camellia sinensis*) leaf (or nettle (*Urtica dioica*) leaf for a caffeine-free option)

1 tsp bilberry (*Vaccinium myrtillus*) berry

½ tsp ginger (*Zingiber officinale*) rhizome

½ tsp fennel (*Foeniculum vulgare*) seed

8 fl oz (240 mL) water

DIRECTIONS

Place herbs in a heat-safe container.

Pour freshly boiled hot water over the herbs, cover, and steep for 20 minutes.

Strain the infusion through a tea strainer and compost or discard plant material.

Serve and enjoy!

Drink up to two servings per day.

Sipping a cup of tea allows us to pause for a moment. Within that pause is the opportunity for stillness and quiet to nourish our mind, body, and spirit.

HERBAL ACADEMY

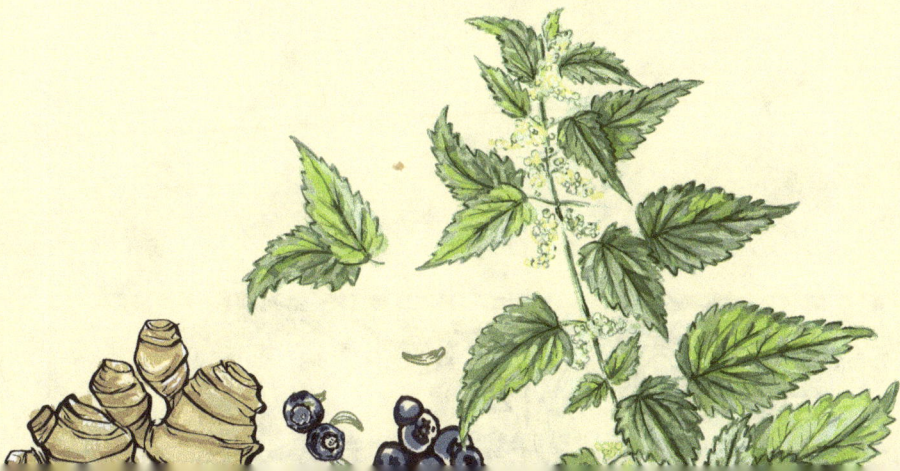

CHAPTER SEVEN
NOT-JUST-FOR-DRINKING TEAS

While botanical teas are most often enjoyed steaming in a mug or chilled in a tall glass over ice, we'd be doing them a disservice if we limited them to drinking alone! As a water-based extraction, herbal teas can be utilized in other ways as we tend to our bodies with water-based therapeutic techniques. In this chapter, we'll share several uses for teas that don't involve drinking—from washes and baths to gargles and compresses—for first aid, skin and hair, or a relaxing, decadent soak.

From top to toe, you'll enjoy botanical hair teas, a flowery facial toner, a gentle mouthwash for tender tissues, a soothing gargle for throat irritation, washes for skin wounds, a soothing herbal sitz bath, a whole-body bath to soak your cares away, and a footbath to keep you dancing through your days. Lean in to the ways herbs can support your whole body, from the outside in!

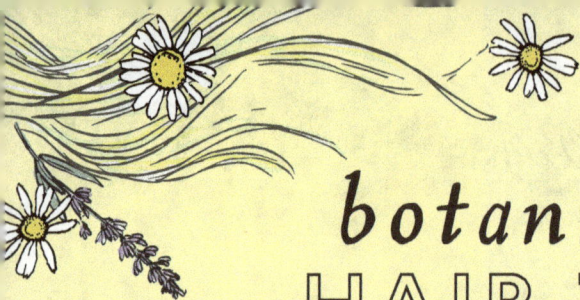

botanical
HAIR TEA

Give your locks a botanical boost with these herbal hair rinses (sans vinegar) to support strength, shine, and a healthy scalp.

Yield: 8 fl oz

INGREDIENTS

Light Hair:

2 tbsp chamomile (*Matricaria chamomilla*) flower

1 tbsp lavender (*Lavandula* spp.) flower bud

8 fl oz (240 mL) water

Dark Hair:

2 tbsp nettle (*Urtica dioica*) leaf

1 tbsp rosemary (*Salvia rosmarinus*) leaf

8 fl oz (240 mL) water

DIRECTIONS

Place herbs in a heat-safe mug or container.

Pour freshly boiled hot water over the herbs, cover, and steep for 20 minutes.

Strain the infusion through a tea strainer and compost or discard plant material.

When tea is at a suitable temperature, pour over hair as the last step of your shower routine.

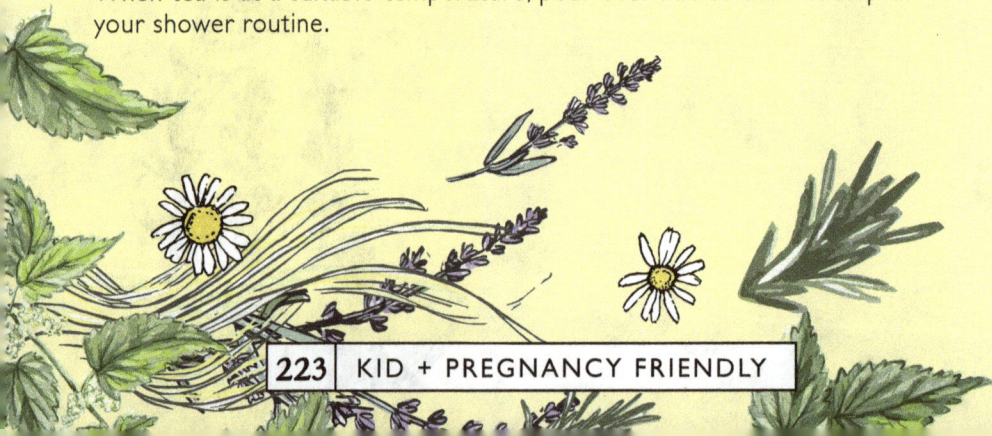

Footloose FOOT SOAK

Our feet carry us through life with the weight of our worlds on them, and after a long day, tension can build up in our feet causing pain and discomfort. As a thank you to these important parts, we can relax them with this tension-reducing herbal foot soak.

Yield: 2 cups dried tea blend

INGREDIENTS

½ cup catnip (*Nepeta cataria*) leaf

½ cup chamomile (*Matricaria chamomilla*) flower

½ cup cramp bark (*Viburnum opulus*) bark

½ cup comfrey (*Symphytum officinale*) leaf

DIRECTIONS

Combine all ingredients and store the blend in a labeled, tightly sealed storage container. Use within 12 months.

Place ½ cup herb blend in a heat-safe container.

Pour 16 fl oz (480 mL) freshly boiled hot water over the herbs, cover, and steep for 30 minutes.

Strain the infusion through a tea strainer and compost or discard plant material.

Transfer liquid to a foot soaking tub and top off with enough warm water to make a comfortable herbal foot bath.

Soak for 15 minutes or as long as it feels good to you.

SOOTHING
Herbal Sitz Bath

A warm herbal bath is a wonderful way to relax the body and the mind post birth. As the physical body enjoys the soothing properties of the herbs, the mind can absorb the calming aroma of the botanicals. This herbal sitz bath is a great gift idea for a new mother.

Yield: 1 cup dried tea blend

INGREDIENTS

¼ cup yarrow (*Achillea millefolium*) aerial parts

¼ cup calendula (*Calendula officinalis*) flower

¼ cup lavender (*Lavandula* spp.) flower bud

2 tbsp witch hazel (*Hamamelis virginiana*) leaf, bark, or twig

2 tbsp rose (*Rosa* spp.) petal

DIRECTIONS

Combine all ingredients and store the blend in a labeled, tightly sealed storage container. Use within 12 months.

Steep 1 cup of tea blend per 64 fl oz (1.9 L) freshly boiled hot water in a heat-safe container, covered, for 30 minutes.

Strain infusion through a tea strainer and compost or discard plant material.

Transfer liquid to the bathtub or sitz bath and top off with enough warm water to make a comfortable herbal sitz bath.

Sore Throat
BOTANICAL GARGLE

Have a sore throat that is bothering you? Whether it's from an allergy-related cough, a viral illness, or cheering too loudly for your favorite team, this botanical gargle can help soothe and bring comfort to throat tissues so you can feel better soon.

Yield: 8 fl oz

INGREDIENTS

1 tbsp peppermint (*Mentha x piperita*) leaf

1 tbsp mullein (*Verbascum thapsus*) leaf

1 tsp licorice (*Glycyrrhiza glabra*) root

8 fl oz (240 mL) water

½ tsp salt

DIRECTIONS

Place herbs in a heat-safe container.

Pour freshly boiled hot water over the herbs, cover, and steep for 10 minutes.

Strain the infusion through a tea strainer lined with an unbleached coffee filter to ensure the removal of tiny mullein leaf hairs, which can cause irritation, and compost or discard plant material.

Add salt, and stir well to combine.

Once tea is comfortably cooled so as not too hot for throat tissues, gargle with a small amount of liquid, spitting liquid out after each gargle. Continue until all liquid has been used, and repeat as often as needed.

Use within 24 hours after straining, if refrigerated.

Use up to 4 times per day.

KID + PREGNANCY FRIENDLY

STRESS-BE-GONE
herbal bath

This soothing herbal bath blend features chamomile, lavender, and linden flower to help ease feelings of stress and melt away the tensions of life. Go ahead and treat yourself. You deserve it!

Yield: 64 fl oz

INGREDIENTS

¼ cup chamomile (*Matricaria chamomilla*) flower

¼ cup lavender (*Lavandula* spp.) flower

¼ cup linden (*Tilia* spp.) flower and bract

64 fl oz (1.9 L) water

DIRECTIONS

Place herbs in a heat-safe container.

Pour freshly boiled hot water over the herbs, cover, and steep for 30 minutes.

Strain infusion through a tea strainer and compost or discard plant material.

Transfer liquid to the bathtub, and top off with enough warm water to make a comfortable bath.

Tissue-Soothing
Herbal Mouthwash

This tissue-soothing mouth rinse is a simple preparation that can be used throughout the day to clean debris from the mouth, soothe inflamed or irritated tissue, or encourage regeneration for minor abrasions in the soft tissue of the mouth.

Yield: 1⅝ cups dried tea blend

INGREDIENTS

¾ cup chamomile (*Matricaria chamomilla*) flower

¾ cup calendula (*Calendula officinalis*) flower

2 tbsp licorice (*Glycyrrhiza glabra*) root

DIRECTIONS

Combine all ingredients and store the blend in a labeled, tightly sealed storage container. Use within 12 months.

Steep 1 tbsp of tea blend per 8 fl oz (240 mL) freshly boiled hot water in a heat-safe container, covered, for 15-20 minutes.

Strain infusion through a tea strainer and compost or discard plant material.

Swish a small amount of liquid around in the mouth, spitting liquid out after each swish. Use after meals or as often as needed.

Use within 24 hours after straining, if refrigerated.

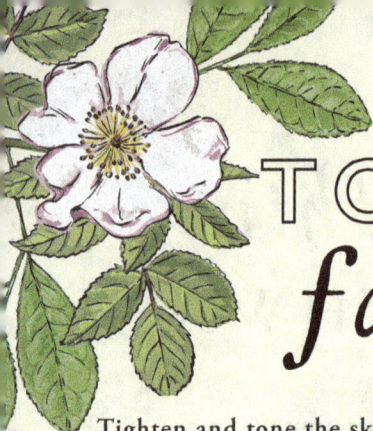

TONE *your* *face* TEA

Tighten and tone the skin on your face while easing inflammation, encouraging even skin tone, and soothing breakouts and irritation with this botanical tea recipe. Use it as the toner step in your morning and evening skin-care regimen and let the astringent, demulcent, and vulnerary properties of this botanical blend support healthy skin.

Yield: 4 fl oz

INGREDIENTS

1 tsp green tea (*Camellia sinensis*) leaf

½ tsp rose (*Rosa* spp.) petal

½ tsp plantain (*Plantago* spp.) leaf

4 fl oz (240 mL) water

DIRECTIONS

Place herbs in a heat-safe container.

Pour freshly boiled hot water over the herbs, cover, and steep for 40 minutes to overnight.

Strain the infusion through a tea strainer and compost or discard plant material.

Use immediately, or within 24 hours after straining, if refrigerated. If desired, freeze extra in an ice cube tray for longer term storage (and an extra cooling application method!).

Apply to skin with a cotton ball or cloth face pad after thoroughly cleansing the skin each morning and evening. Follow up with a moisturizer or nourishing botanical oil.

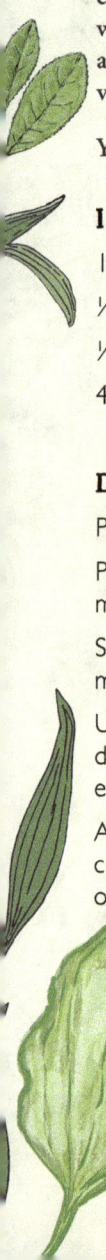

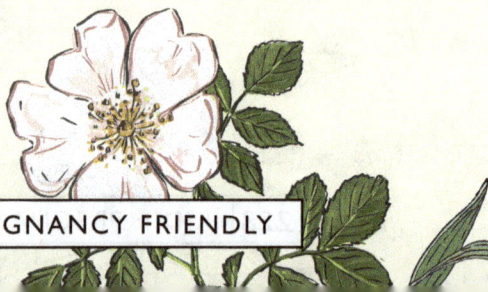

topical tea
Vulnerary Compress

If your tissues need support knitting themselves back into shape, this vulnerary tea blend can do the trick. Simply make this compress blend and then use a washcloth to apply directly to the broken or damaged tissue. You could also choose to use this blend as a soak.

Yield: 8 fl oz

INGREDIENTS

2 tsp plantain (*Plantago* spp.) leaf

I tsp calendula (*Calendula officinalis*) flower

I tsp chamomile (*Matricaria chamomilla*) flower

8 fl oz (240 mL) water

DIRECTIONS

Place herbs in a heat-safe container.

Pour freshly boiled hot water over the herbs, cover, and steep for 10-20 minutes.

Strain the infusion through a tea strainer and compost or discard plant material.

Allow the mixture to cool to a comfortable temperature, soak a washcloth in the tea and apply to tissues.

KID + PREGNANCY FRIENDLY

WOUND
WASH TEA

The first thing to do when you get a wound of any kind is to clean it well before applying other supportive herbal preparations. This wound wash tea is the perfect thing to clean minor cuts, scrapes, bites, and wounds, flushing them of dirt and debris, discouraging microbial growth, and slowing excessive bleeding.

Yield: 8 fl oz

INGREDIENTS

2 tsp yarrow (*Achillea millefolium*) aerial parts

1 tsp calendula (*Calendula officinalis*) flower

1 tsp lavender (*Lavandula* spp.) flower bud

8 fl oz (240 mL) water

DIRECTIONS

Place herbs in a heat-safe container.

Pour freshly boiled hot water over the herbs, cover, and steep for 10-20 minutes.

Strain the infusion through a tea strainer and compost or discard plant material.

Allow the mixture to cool to a comfortable temperature and apply to the wound, being sure to thoroughly wash the affected area well. Gently pat dry before applying further herbal preparations to the area.

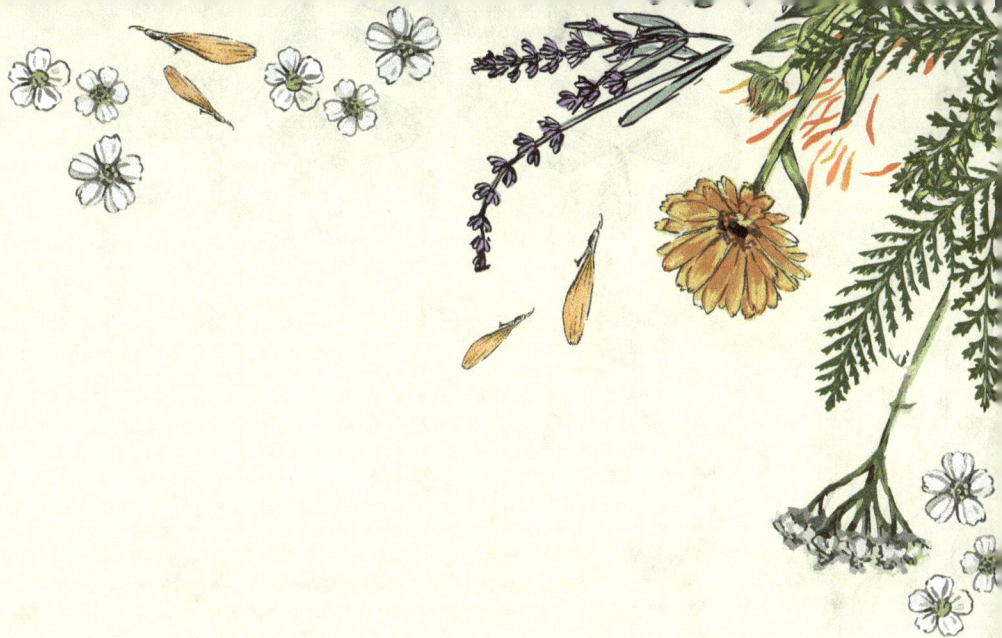

You can sip a cup of homemade herbal tea to help you wake up in the morning, focus in the afternoon, or rest deeper at night. There are brews that help soothe fevers, ease occasional aches and pains, melt away daily stresses, and even nurture a grieving heart.

HERBAL ACADEMY

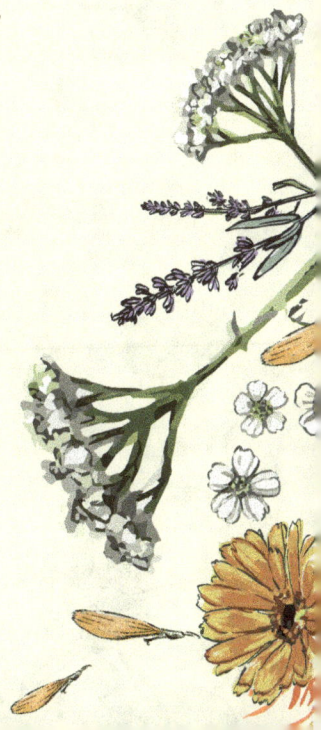

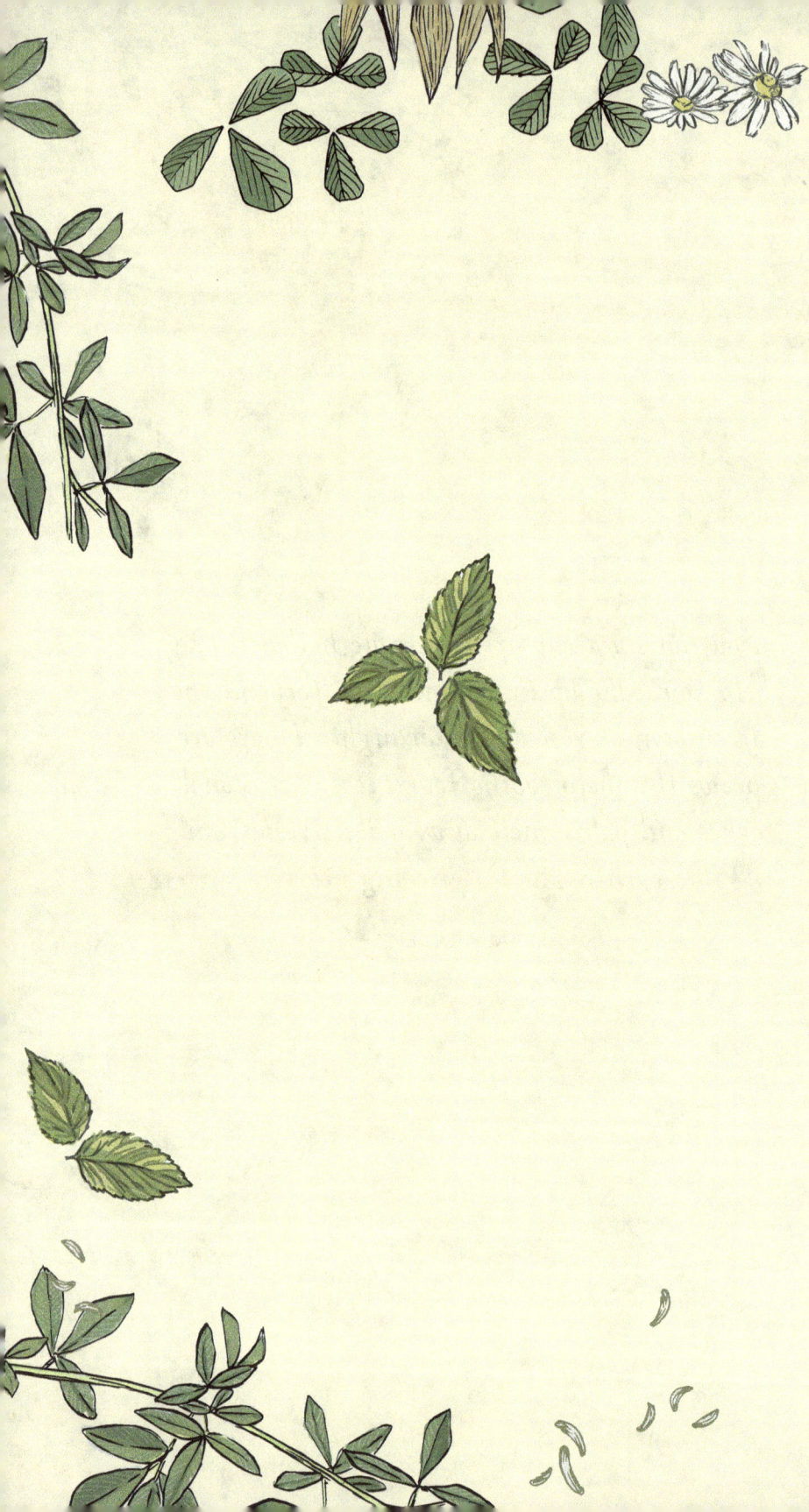

CHAPTER EIGHT
CHEERS!

Thank you for joining us for tea time and bringing these botanical tea blend recipes into your own herbal practice!

We are enthralled by the beauty, the countless unique flavors, the perfectly balancing energetics, and the immeasurable benefits of herbs and herbal tea blends and feel so grateful to have the opportunity to weave them into our lives in delicious ways. From greeting the day with Tulsi Sunrise Tea and chilling out with Cool Off Minty Sun Tea, to sipping Gentle Digestive Tea as an after-dinner accompaniment and peacefully finding slumber with Midwinter Night's Dream Tea, botanical tea blends meet us where we are and so often provide just what's needed in the moment.

What are you needing—today or this season? Perhaps you'd like to have certain blends on hand to help you address acute concerns, or maybe you'd like to savor the ritual of making herbal tea to help you tune in to seasonal rhythms. There are so many reasons to enjoy botanical tea blends, and we hope this recipe book has given you many, many options and ideas to do just that.

Are you inspired and ready to learn more about making your own tea blends that taste delicious and are tailored to support your unique physical and emotional needs? This recipe book grew out of our desire to help more folks build confidence brewing up herbal tea in their own kitchens, and started with the 12 botanical tea blends we included in our **Tea Blending 101 Mini Course**.

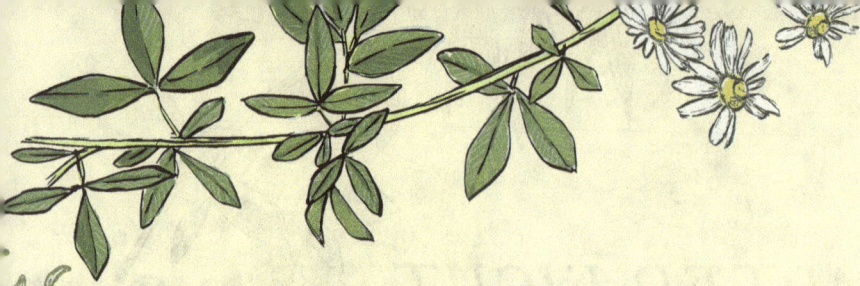

This hands-on course walks you through an easy-to-follow process of choosing herbs to formulate safe blends that are pleasing to the senses and have a positive impact on the whole person. In fact, it is built around 12 tea-friendly common herbs (with suggestions for substitutes) to help you hone in on your tea-blending skills. If you're ready to graduate to this next step and fall in love with tea blending, we invite you to join us in class!

Explore all of our courses and workshops at *theherbalacademy.com*

We'd love for you to connect with us in our vibrant online community, visiting us at the platforms below and sharing the tea recipes you make by tagging us in your post or using the hashtag #myherbalstudies.

INSTAGRAM
@HERBALACADEMY

FACEBOOK
@THEHERBALACADEMY

PINTEREST
@THEHERBALACADEMY

YOUTUBE
@HERBALACADEMY

Sip, sip hooray from your friends and educators at the Herbal Academy!

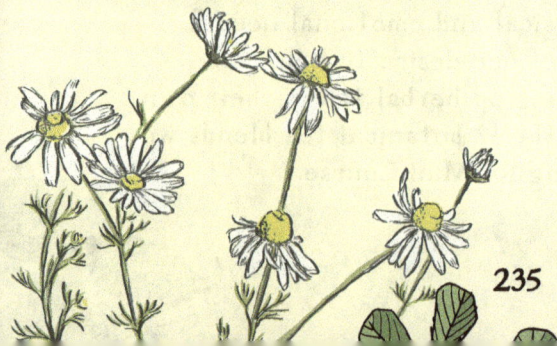

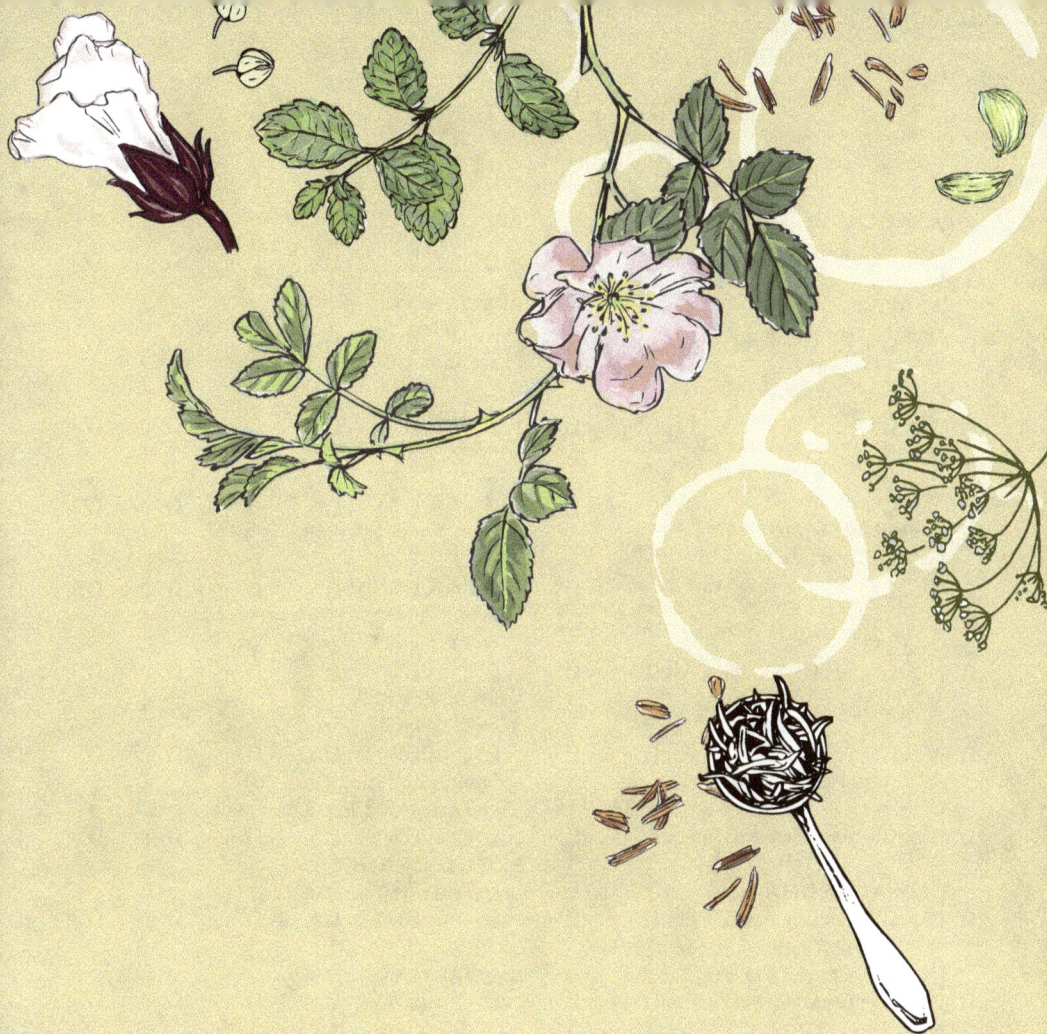

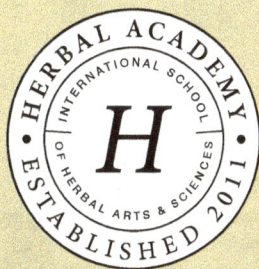

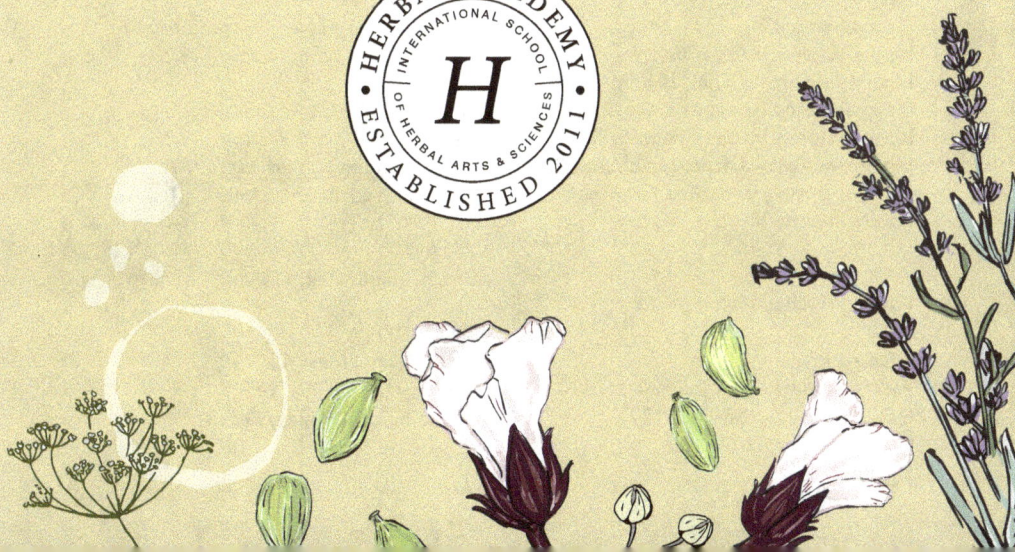

INDEX

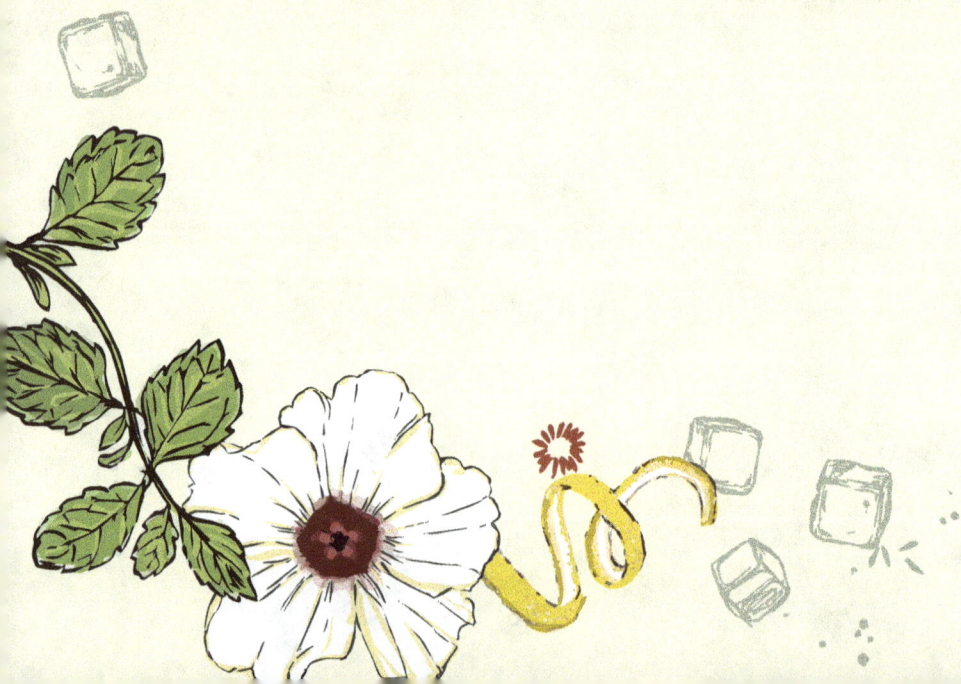

LINE YOUR BOOKSHELF WITH THE ENTIRE HERBAL ACADEMY BOTANICAL RECIPE BOOK COLLECTION!

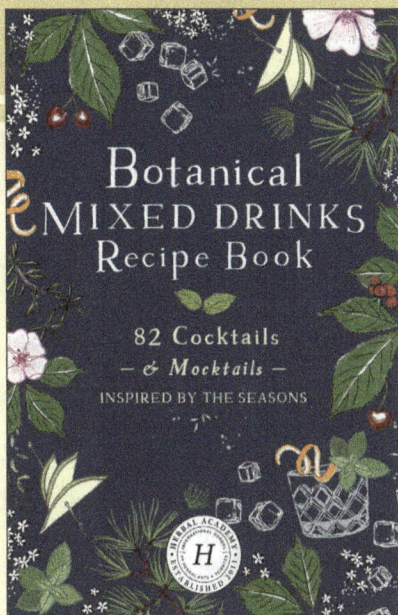

Botanical MIXED DRINKS Recipe Book

82 Cocktails
— & Mocktails —
INSPIRED BY THE SEASONS

Botanical SKIN CARE Recipe Book

Featuring 194
favorite tried-and-tested
herbal skin care recipes!

4.8 STARS on Amazon!

With our penchant for soothing herbal teas, refreshing botanical shrubs, warming winter cocoas, and tasty before-dinner apéritifs, it's safe to say herbalists know drinks!

The *Botanical Mixed Drinks Recipe Book* infuses herbal whimsy into 82 flavorful botanical cocktails and mocktails, shares step-by-step guidance for crafting a well-stocked herbal bar, and enchants beginner and sage mixologists with an inspiring, functional keepsake collection.

BUY THESE BOOKS ON THE HERBAL ACADEMY WEBSITE,

theherbalacademy.com

AMAZON, BARNES & NOBLE, INDIE BOUND, AND OTHER BOOKSTORES.

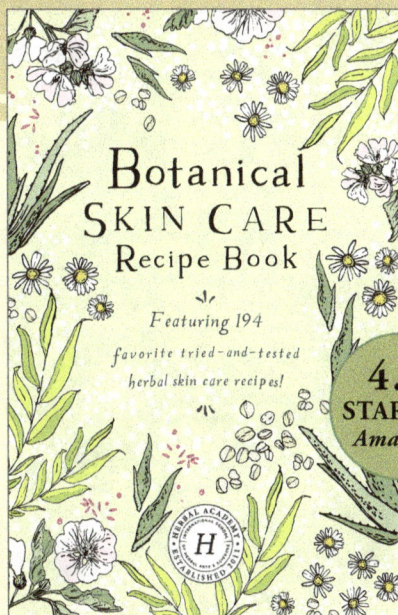

When it comes to our wellbeing and the health of the largest organ in our bodies—our skin—we have the opportunity to design a skin care regimen that addresses our unique needs!

The 194 recipes provided in this book are curated from the Herbal Academy's Botanical Skin Care Course, so you can feel confident knowing that these skin care products are safe, effective, and well-loved and used by our team of herbalists! Ditch the store-bought, questionable bottles lining your bathroom closet—the *Botanical Skin Care Recipe Book* makes it possible for you to easily prepare your own skin care products right at home.

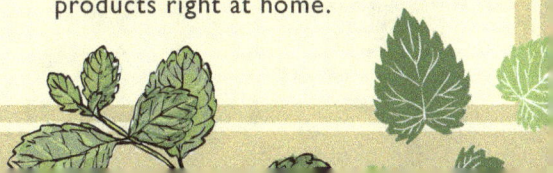